full exposure

full **exposure**

opening up to sexual creativity
and erotic expression

susie bright

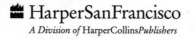
HarperSanFrancisco
A Division of HarperCollins*Publishers*

HarperCollins books may be purchased for educational, business, or sales promotional use. For information please write: Special Markets Department, HarperCollins Publishers, 10 East 53rd Street, New York, NY 10022.

HarperCollins Web Site: http://www.harpercollins.com

HarperCollins®, 📖 ®, and HarperSanFrancisco™ are trademarks of Harper-Collins Publishers Inc.

FIRST EDITION

Designed by Laura Lindgren and Celia Fuller

Library of Congress Cataloging-in-Publication Data
Bright, Susie.
    Full exposure : opening up to sexual creativity and erotic expression /
Susie Bright. — 1st ed.
        p.   cm.
    ISBN 0—06—251554—3 (cloth)
    ISBN 0—06—251591—8 (paper)
    1. Sex (psychology) I. Title. II. Title: Opening up to sexual creativity
and erotic expression.
    BF692.B746 1999   99—23097
    306.7—dc21

99 00 01 02 03 ❖RRD(H) 10 9 8 7 6 5 4 3 2 1

acknowledgments

I'd like to thank all the people who helped me write this book: my partner, Jon Bailiff; my father, Bill Bright; my managers, Jo-Lynne Worley and Joanie Shoemaker; and my editors, Mark Chimsky and Doug Abrams. I am grateful to my mother, Elizabeth Bright, and my daughter, Aretha Bright, for all their support. Many thanks also to my secretary, Jennifer Taillac, who was of great assistance to me. And in the inspiration department, thank you to Michael Anderson, Kim Anno, Helen Behar, Alex Conn, Honey Lee Cottrell, Gosnell Duncan, Jennie Giammasi, Alicia Goldberg, Rebecca Hall, Joe Mancino, Jenni Olsen, Shar Rednour, Jared Rutter, Lana Sandahl, David Steinberg, and Carter Wilson.

For Jon

contents

full exposure

opening up

There is no such thing as a person without an erotic story. I don't mean a tall tale or a punch line or a story about the one who got away. I'm talking about a personal erotic identity, what you might call a sexual philosophy. It's the big "What If?" of our sexual lives.

Take a look at your own erotic story, and you'll see that it's a motion picture of everything about you that is creative: the risks you'd be willing to take, the weightless depth of your imagination, your attraction to the truth, and the things that would make you go blind. That's a story all right. It doesn't matter whether we tell it to a crowd of thousands, whisper it to our lover, or merely confess it to ourselves. The power is in owning it.

In this book, I want to cut through all the labels and politics and reveal what I've learned about sex—what has been transformative for me as a lover, a parent, a daughter, and an artist. I want to argue that sexuality is the soul of the creative process and that erotic expression of any kind is a personal revolution.

Let me propose my erotic manifesto to you—a message for lovers who want to express their minds and bodies without a border between the two—who sense that their erotic notions are more than just masturbation candy. I want to connect with people who live, make love, nurture, battle, dream, sing, and sacrifice with the sense that sex is more than just flesh, but hardly an ethereal affair.

Sex is known to everyone as the seed of our physical creation. But we don't often recognize, or even admit, that it's also the wellspring of our creativity. How many people are willing to name their erotic character as one of their most demanding or enlightening teachers? If you want to be a student of sexual life, or a teacher, plenty of questions need to be asked first:

- Why is it so threatening to address sexual desire consciously in the first place?

- What will everyone say about you when you do "come out of the closet" erotically?

- How can parents ever be seen by their kids as real sexual people without violating the boundaries of their nurturing relationship?

- What are the real—and fake—differences between men and women's sense of the erotic?

- Is the best erotic expression soulful? Does it have a spiritual or philosophical embrace? Or is that just romantic drivel?

- How do talking, reading, and writing about sex affect your actual sex life?

- What's the point in discussing something in public that's so innately private?

- For the last fucking time, is there a difference between erotica and pornography?

- Why does our very language seem so inadequate for talking about our sexual feelings and behavior?

- Is there such a thing as "sex jag"?

- Who are the best lovers, anyway? Can one even make that kind of judgment?

- What does erotic expression teach us about our bodies?

- Is there a line to be drawn in erotic creativity? Can you go too far?

- Finally, how can articulate erotic expression make us better lovers, or even better people?

Every time I've been changed by reading a book, it was because the authors asked me the right questions. The writer drew me the outline of a picture and left me to my own colorful revelations. Now, as I sit down to write this book, the picture I want to draw encompasses my whole lifetime of sex, and for once, I'll say it: I have an agenda. I've wiped the question mark off my face. I think it's natural, in our current circumstances, to feel desperate or cynical about sex. Of course we don't start out that way . . . but information is scarce, and prejudice is overabundant. In our efforts to be honest or realistic about sex, we often can't even get past the naked basics.

But this book isn't about the physical. There will be no dia-grams—and zero about technique. This book is about the personal meaning of erotic expression: the creativity it demands, the challenges of sexual candor, and the rewards of coming clean about desire. It's there, in that story of the lover's mind and body, that I've set my lens to a full exposure.

chapter two

Nothing really exists except examples.
Wittgenstein

If I had to judge my sex life by how many times I jump into bed and have an orgasm, I'd get a big fat *F*. Oh, I'm sure my notches are more than someone else's notches, but I've had long, medium, and short stretches of time in my life where I haven't buttered up to anybody else's body, or even had my own private Jill-off.

Yet this is the last thing I think of when I consider my erotic life. I say "erotic life" instead of "sex life," because when someone asks me about my *sex* life, it's like code for, "Are you getting laid?" I need a code for replying, "Getting laid isn't the half of it." My dreams are filled with sex; my work is inspired with sexual energy; my family and friendships are influenced in so many ways by my sexual creativity that I couldn't even pinpoint them all. Most sex experts tell people to search for a sex life, to make it happen by getting out of the house and into the right singles bar, but actually your sex life is rocking your boat every minute of every day. You never even have to leave the house or make a phone call.

I remember snooping in a neighbor's bookshelves when I was a kid, discovering their garishly illustrated *Kama Sutra* technique manual with more than a hundred pages and a hundred pretzel shapes to screw your body into. It had all the appeal of a periodic table. *This* is what I had to learn to have sex? It was a strangely unemotional examination. The book's title invoked erotic and spiritual symbols—but the spirit behind the presentation was chopped liver. I had been so excited to think that one day I was going to have a sex life, a real adult sex life—and I imagined it would be as exciting and inspiring as the sexy music I heard on the radio, the romantic novels I read, or the passionate embraces I saw dissolve on the movie screens.

My childhood intuition was right. Those top-forty hits I heard on the radio were more sexy than a hundred nudist diagrams. Rock 'n' roll *was* sex, and so were all those novels and movies I thrilled to—because those things actually possessed sexual creativity, and the people who composed them were probably as inspired as I was when they first came up with their ideas.

Erotic experience is a wake-up call; it's the sign that you're not only alive, you're bursting. As my friend Michael once said, "It doesn't matter whether you're cooking a meal, or playing a game of basketball, or writing a chapter. Sometimes you get this rush of holistic energy, and you'd swear that you just got laid."

"I know that," I told him, "but how come more people won't admit it? It's not like I can line up a row of architects and rocket scientists to admit that, yes indeed, "they split that atom, they built that bridge," and they owe it all to some serious erotic inspiration. Everyone thinks that if they admit how much sexual energy fuels their everyday life and accomplishments, they won't get any respect."

"But it doesn't matter what they say!" Michael is very good at overriding all naysayers. "Haven't they ever heard of a little thing called sublimation? Dr. Freud, hello! You go to any museum, you look at the classic Renaissance paintings, where everyone is supposed to be praising God and fearing the devil, but what is it, after all? Naked bodies everywhere! You're going to tell me these painters didn't get off on that? Their faith, their painting, their sexual energy—it's all the same thing."

People often don't want to hear that their religious feeling is erotic; it's an insult to them. They take the holier-than-thou attitude that any kind of scholarship, any kind of profession or art, needs to be unsullied by sex in order to be worthy.

But what is their worthiness all about? Michael started in describing Dante's *Divine Comedy*. "Here we have a hero who goes from hell to purgatory to paradise, and at the end of it all— after he has seen God—what does he say? He speaks out to the memory of one woman, a woman he saw for only an instant, and she is 'the love that moves the sun and all the stars!' Remember, this is *after* God!"

"Yes, I think of that quote, 'God is in the details,' " I said. "And so is sex."

Your erotic life is what you notice about yourself—what drives you and thrills you and even maroons you sometimes. It influences our every personal expression, our role models, and the picture of our generation. I can read poems I wrote as a teenager, look at the image of myself giving birth to my daughter ten years ago, or see myself on a stage today—and an erotic thread runs through all of it. My character shows how motivated

I've been by sexual creativity, long before I knew much at all about "having sex."

I don't have to visit a museum or look at the classics to see how sex and art intersect from the moment we pick up our pen or our brush. I used to visit my friend Kimi in her art studio, where she made huge abstract expressionist paintings, from floor to ceiling. She routinely had her vibrator plugged in, lying on the rug next to her latest canvas, along with her brushes, rags, and colors. She caught me looking at it one day, and she said, "I can't help it, I get so excited sometimes! And other times I'm so tired, this is the only thing that gets me going again."

People have long debated whether eroticism saps their energy or lets it fly. A physical orgasm can sometimes make you so weak in the knees that you feel closer to a nap than to creating a masterpiece. But that's why it's so important to see the difference between the release of an orgasm and the release of the creative sexual mind.

A fantasy never leaves you exhausted, an erotic inspiration never tires you out. Erotic inspiration can be released through orgasms—but that's just one way. More important is that sexual creativity stems from living life as if you were making something of it—instead of being made over. I'm not talking about denying physical release, or saving your jizz up like some precious reservoir. No, I mean the way we express the juice of our greatest joys, and some of the most righteous justice in our lives. Why don't we recognize the erotic element in that passion?

We are burdened by assumptions that sex is the dirtiest thing you can do. People go miles out of their way to defend their artistic and intellectual intentions by saying, "This work is not about sex." That's how you're supposed to be able to tell how grand and incredible it all is—that it's *not* sexual. If it's real love, then it's not about sex. If it's real art, it's not about sex. If it's real politics . . .

When people put faith, scholarship, and science in front of their sexual creativity like a large, impenetrable screen, then look at what they're hiding. They are trying to hide the power of sex, as if a lot of colorful denunciations could make it go away. They are chained to their superstitious fears about sexual power instead of embracing its potential—a place of enormous opportunity, yet incredible insecurities.

I don't blame our ancestors for being as afraid of sex as they were. When I think of my own mother telling me that as a teenager in puberty she had no idea why she started bleeding— not even knowing the word *menstruation*—then I think about how much of our lives have been spent being terrified of our bodies. We are mystified by the origins of life and causes of death—sensing the sexual connection but feeling utterly helpless to control its consequences or causes.

Even though so much of our ignorance is in the past and our physical bodies are more revealed and understood every day, the odd thing is that the scientific revolution has not entirely made a sexual revolution. A true sexual revolution would bring about a change of consciousness, increasing our scientific knowledge a hundredfold. Nowadays, there's probably not a single American woman my age who doesn't understand what menstruation means—but are there women who nevertheless are utterly mystified about every other aspect of their genitals? Yes, I know hundreds. They know all about tampons, but they have no clue about their sexual nature. Men are hardly better off. Do most men feel like they understand the connection between their erotic mind and their body's response? Hardly. When we do get a clue about what makes us tick, we're more than likely to get a shaming lecture from someone who claims we shouldn't have been thinking about it in the first place.

I got a letter just the other day from some outraged citizen wagging his finger at me. This particular man wrote, "Susie, you don't know what LOVE is. Love is not sex. It's about trust, it's about sacrifice, it's about something that lasts."

Well, I don't know what awful experiences this man has had with his body and his desires. Maybe someday he'll realize that sexual feeling is so lasting that you experience it from cradle to grave. Sex does demand a humility that comes only with the deepest sacrifices. Sex is one of the few honest places inside us; it doesn't know how to lie, even if we change the story for the public.

Sex is not about whatever woman done him wrong or about some one-night stand he'll always regret. It's first and always about the capacity to create and feel, and express and connect. You can certainly love without fucking, but I don't think anyone loves without an element of erotic tenderness, anxiety, and a sense of wonder. If erotic life is really something larger than a carnal life or sexual gymnastics, then it doesn't really matter whether you're a porn star or a virgin—your erotic comprehension is about being alive—and feeling something that makes you bigger than the sometimes ugly circumstances of our existence would ever let us believe.

It's not an original idea that sex and creativity are connected or that sexual inspiration opens a path of consciousness and strength that otherwise may be elusive. It's just that we don't always find enlightenment at the end of all our sexual pursuits. At the end of the sexual seeker's journey, there sometimes seems to be an erotic whoopee cushion, the indignity and humiliation of a lustful quest gone wrong. How many times have we shaken our heads at our folly? How often does a sexual high come down like a bad acid hangover?—I thought I saw God, but it was really a pimple on my ass.

Erotic hindsight is more than just one sorry individual's humiliations and regrets. Whole groups of seekers have felt that there had to be more to sexual and creative success than the pain of individual trial and error. Maybe there was a guru or a new kind of faith that could lead us out of the erotic wilderness! I've met the enlightenment escapees, who typically gather around one central figure, the fearless leader with a direct line to nirvana. He—and it's always a he—is the quintessential phallocrat to whom every member must submit. Somehow the sexism of this tradition impresses me more than the sex. I've never heard of a cult where everyone had to worship the leader's clitoris.

The problem is that most of the New Age has examined the sexual prejudices of its faith just as poorly as any traditional religion. When sects pursue doctrine at the expense of contradictions—when they turn insights into delusions of superiority, or inspirations into idols—they're never going to get to the wellspring of sexual energy. Sexual honesty, let alone creativity, will never flourish among the conformists or the elitists. We need something bigger, much bigger, to accommodate the spectrum of our erotic imaginations.

When people feel sullied by their passion, they often try to take the sex out of it, as if sex were the root of corruption. They find it easier to talk about the greater glory of eros if they keep it cosmic, out of gender, ahistorical, bathed in fairy tales and pink lights. I like dancing in a fairy ring under a rosy spotlight as much as the next person, but I can't accept the phoniness of a full-time, think-pink lifestyle. Eros *is* in the details, but those finer senses can bloom anywhere.

I've come to my own understanding of sexual creativity with plenty of hindsight. I've felt desire make a fool of me, I've followed various characters I had the hots for as if they held my soul in their hands, I've vowed to remove myself from the fleshly indignities that made me feel low—especially after my soul got handed back to me with a few holes in it.

I once loved a man who everyone, including the man himself, told me was bad news. He drove me crazy. Just recently, after years of little contact with him, he called me up to say he was splitting town, and he asked me to store a trunk of his personal belongings. He dropped off the trunk and told me I might get a kick out of what was inside. He didn't give me any details, and now I know why. That trunk was filled with hundreds of letters from every woman he's known in the past forty years, accusing him of ripping their hearts out and just plain ruining their lives. I'm awfully nosy, but reading even one of those letters was so painful that I just had to close the lid after a few minutes.

When I was in love with him, so many years ago, I tried to think up all sorts of "respectable" reasons for why he was worth loving, but I had to admit that my fever for him was 99.9 percent inspired by a sexual craving that seemed out of control. Even then, I could see that the experience of making love with him was not nearly as good as the yearning for it. It was like being hungry for food. My friends gave me the usual rap—you know, women who love assholes, loving what you can't have, breaking the pattern, blah blah blah. But I didn't have a pattern. I had never felt anything like this before. I enjoyed the love of many who were decent, kind, and faithful. But that didn't make a dent in what I was feeling for this lover.

What seemed critical at the time was whether or not I saw him, whether or not I touched him. But I was missing the point.

Something about meeting him at the time I did was like a thunderclap; it awakened a part of my erotic spirit that I was totally unacquainted with.

In all the fracas about what a bastard he was and how I had played the hapless victim, I never took stock of how I'd gained access to sexual feelings I'd never had before. No matter what happened to him, I was never going to lose this knowledge. I had more empathy, more passion, more patience, and a whole new take on surrender. This power had always been inside me; the cork couldn't have stayed in too much longer. His caress or the smell of his room or the way the light hit me the day we met—which catalyst would I make my offering to? I'm thankful that I woke up at all.

I don't like to strike a redemptive pose—how you first have to crawl through my mud before you can sit smug at the top. I'm writing this book more to reach out to every person who ever thought, "There's more to sex than anyone admits." I want to tell them how much I agree and how much we could increase the richness of this realization if we didn't try to excuse it or hide it or give it another name. It's not just time for admission, it's time for respect.

We have no tradition in our culture for showing respect to anything sexual. We don't promote erotic education. Our health care establishment barely has a clue about our sexual bodies. Our political system finds sex to be a fine whipping boy. The gossips and preachers are our typical sex advisers, and their tone is usually damning, rarely daring.

So how does anyone dare? When I do feel at ease about sex, or blunt or curious, then the rewards are so immediate and obvious that it's a great incentive to do it again. The ease just comes with familiarity. I've probably listened to others tell me about their sex lives more than I've talked about my own, and hearing their stories influences my advice more than anything else.

I've been guilty myself of trying to fix my friends' sex problems with surefire remedies before I ever heard them say what they wanted in the first place. I've sent my favorite vibrator, festooned with a red bow, to a girlfriend who I thought was in need, only to have her ship it back with a note that said, "Does *nothing* for me." I've shown my favorite porn film to an audience of serious erotica scholars, only to have them critique it as everything from "way too violent" to "an existentialist homage" to "pretty fucking hot except for that fat guy in the double penetration scene."

Clearly, guidelines for erotic living have to avoid matters of taste. First, we have to resist the urge to pathologize everyone's sex life. The puritans are suspicious of sex education because it leads to tolerance, and there's a world of sexual learning in everything from anatomy books to *Leaves of Grass* to *Hot Legs* magazine. I used to be embarrassed that my sex knowledge came more from books than from experience, but by the time my experience caught up with my library, I could say that a great book was on a par with a great fuck, without disrespect to the lessons learned from either.

Tolerance and knowledge are the preconditions for candor. I was asked last year to teach a class about lesbian and gay social issues, substituting for a couple of teachers who had taught the course for years. One of their most effective exercises for their students was to ask them to write a hypothetical coming-out letter to their parents, friends, or work mates. I was struck by this gay phrase, since *coming out*—used in times past only by debutantes—has a much bigger definition now that we know how demanding any sexual identity can be. Gay? Lesbian? That's not the half of it! People make fun of organizations with names like "Gay-Bisexual-Lesbian-Transgendered-or-Wondering," and the "wonder" part is really the most psychologically astute. We are all in a state of wonder about who we are sexually. I want to ask my new students to investigate what "coming out" means, not by the crudest labels, but when sexuality is truly individual.

Take, for example, the student whose mom is a lesbian—a mom who expected her child to be heterosexual and was well prepared for that eventuality. When her daughter says instead that she's a lesbian, too, but not the kind of dyke her mom was, her mom explodes. Daughter likes S/M, mother spits up her granola. What does *coming out* mean in their family?

Another case from my classrooms: a passionate, feminist man hides his porn collection from his girlfriend, because he thinks it's a contradiction that neither she nor he can accept in public. Little does he know that his girlfriend, the one he thinks is so righteous, has been having sex for years without a single orgasm, though she has convinced all her lovers otherwise. Now she would like to confide in her boyfriend, but she fears a loss of sexual power if she reveals herself. When are they going to *come out* to each other?

Or how about the gay man in my class who was the center of gay politics on campus, yet confided in his journal that he'd had bisexual fantasies all his life? He might have something to share with the heterosexual man in the same room who reveals that his constant lesbian fantasies are vicarious, not something he'd like to step into as a man.

All these people have an urgent coming-out letter in the making. Mere homosexuality can just get in line with every other erotic stripe. I used to think it was only gay people who were crowding up the closet, but now it's clear to me that it is the overgeneralized "heterosexuals" who need to speak up for them-selves. You've seen the T-shirt: "I'm Straight but Not Narrow." That's an open invitation to give up on the labels and try some-thing a little more personal.

"What am I to say?—Everyone is gay," Kurt Cobain wrote in one of his most-quoted lyrics. His tone of voice—"Can you please get over yourselves?"—caught a feeling that was in the air for many people. Whatever you "are," you are first of all a sexual person who has a limitless mind. Why keep up the pretense?

We've all heard the gay celebrities' testimonies about how good it feels "not to lie anymore," how they avoided or overcame a nervous breakdown by coming clean with their sex story. What about everyone else, what are they waiting for? I'd give anything to hear some high-profile heterosexual Hollywood couple go on the record that they choose not to be monogamous, or that they read erotic stories to each other, or that they think biological gender is overrated.

Someday sexual "orientation" is going to bust open, just as notions of "race" have been torn apart in recent years, and it will become clear to everyone that we've only made these stupid cat-egories so that some people could fancy themselves superior to others. "Coming out" applies to all of us. This very personal sword of truth slices through the knotted vines that have choked off our erotic development. The hardest part of it is knowing yourself well enough to make the first cut.

big enough

When I was a kid, I would ask older friends—the baby-sitters, the playground divas—to tell me everything they knew about sex. I wanted to know what the four-letter words meant, what the jokes were about, how the rules operated. The big girls informed me that sex was a terribly big deal but that I was too little to understand it. They said I didn't know how to "do it," that it was way beyond my body and over my head. Too bad I didn't know the word *orgasm* at the time, or I could have mentioned that I was having some of them. Maybe that would have cracked their smug exteriors.

By the time I was a young adult, I had the idea that I was "big enough" to do it, but now, because of the combination of wrong genes and lost opportunities, I was unfit for seduction. No one was ever going to want me, I wasn't beautiful, I wasn't powerful, I didn't have enough *gain*. I still didn't understand half the dirty jokes.

Finally, someone came along, and I did do it. I remember going to school the next day, euphoric but amazed, like I was wearing a special pair of glasses that could look into every other teenager's sex history. I peered at everyone trudging toward the bell and whispered, "Why was I ever bamboozled by this? I thought everyone was in the golden circle except me." But I could see, from the look in their eyes, how practically everyone on campus was as small and lonely as I had been the week before. It was one dirty joke all right. When I recognized the same loneliness in some of the teachers' eyes as well, I realized that my afterglow bubble wasn't going to last.

What's so strange about those "first times," and other conquests is that they never seem to give you any security for the future. I eventually went back to gnawing on my own paw, an easy prey for jealousy, competition, regrets, and ambivalence. Even when I found one person who wanted me, it offered no solace that this miracle would happen again. I was in that despicable sexual ice cube tray where I thought the only good things that would ever happen to me would be because I got "picked." And it wasn't that I was so passive, either. I just wouldn't cop to the remarkable power I had. I wasn't convinced that I was big enough, so someone else had to be.

How did I ever get to the point of knowing I was attractive enough, worthy and loving enough? It was from listening to my lovers and friends tell their stories. At first, I admit, it was pretty shallow—I just got the biggest kick out of having my body admired. I had always been noticed for being an egghead, and to have puberty transform me into a sex object was like the typical Marian the Librarian taking the pins out of her hair: I'm a goddess *and* a nerd!

At the same time, I noticed that my lovers' impressions of me, at their most poignant and appreciative, didn't come from my being dressed up or at my most self-prepared. If someone adores you when you're down and out, you start to get the idea that your attraction isn't based on a clean shave or the perfect lipstick. The most uninhibited sex I've ever had was not neat and tidy; my orgasm was not a set piece. I know those experiences are not always enough for lovers to feel secure; many keep doubting that anyone wants to be with them, in spite of evidence to the contrary.

In front of me is a current magazine, and in it a famous actress says that not a day goes by when she doesn't wonder what on earth her boyfriend sees in her, since she's not a perfect beauty. It makes me cringe to hear women talk like that! All day people tell her that she's a babe, and every day she receives piles of fan mail from men who'd give anything to be with her. This is in addition to her adoring boyfriend. I don't think the solution lies in one more person telling her, "No, really, you *are* desirable." The remedy for people who feel unlovable is to get off their *toilette* and love someone back. Can Miss Movie Star stop scrutinizing her own belly-button defects long enough to consider how she expresses her own love and desire?

I know that the deeper I have felt desire for another and the more I could express it, the less weight I have put on my own worthiness. Loving other people's flaws has made me a lot less dedicated to my own. At eighteen I may have been in my physical prime, but my erotic life was in its infancy, with its concerns of appearance and worthiness. I was so *surprised* when I fell in love, and surprised at how much I loved to make love, because I had no idea how personal, and chaotic and defiant it could be. Why did I ever think that sexual confidence was something you could buy or put on, something for the perfect ingenue? Sometimes I feel like taking out a mock advertisement that says: *Improve your sex life! Get older!*

I deepened my sexual life, not because my résumé improved, or my vital statistics went up the chart, but because I realized being "good enough" was nothing but a scare tactic. I had everything I needed except the courage to admit that I was the one holding the door, playing with the keys.

When you're born, you're ready for sex. This whole business of being "ready" is strange, because some people are never going to get to the starting line, no matter how many gray hairs they have. And that's such a shame, when we all have bodies that are so ideally sexual to begin with. I remember the old Hollywood romance where the hero gazes upon the damsel in his arms and says, "You were made for love!" Well, really, who isn't? We're accustomed to saying that the only all-accepting love is maternal; we feel pity for people that "only a mother could love." But maternal love is just one facet of erotic love— because it is the erotic imagination and generosity in our spirit that makes such "maternal" sacrifice and unconditional appreciation possible.

Motherhood often gets to stand in as the wholesome face for sexual appreciation and devotion, because it's so much more acceptable to people's idea of the Virgin Mary as the ultimate woman. In fact, childbirth—as I have said since I first went into labor—is the ultimate sex act. I wish I were one of those people who say they can remember being born, but I can only hold on to my memories of being the deliverer. All those hidden parts of my body that I once thought were for pleasure, or had otherwise ignored, suddenly became the center of the universe. From between my legs, like a legend, someone alive and breathing emerged. If having someone make an entrance to the world through your cunt isn't the last word in sexuality, I don't know what is.

Nevertheless, we all arrive erotically perfect. From the moment we respond to a loving touch, we learn to suckle, kiss, and respond to the warmth of a caress and an adoring voice.

Sex actually starts out being big enough for *one:* one person who has a body, enthusiasm, affection, and imagination. Are we big enough to get excited about things, to give and take affection with pleasure? Do we understand, without melodrama, that our genitals are part of our natural body? This is the large place where we want to live.

There are precious few adults in this country who grew up feeling at ease with their genitals or with masturbation or nudity or any other strong solo sex feeling. We all confronted these sensations at some time, and luckily some of us wondered what all the secrecy was about. Our curiosity, rebellion, wonderment—and last but hardly least, our very own sex drive—kept us alive and questioning when almost every adult and institution around us said no.

Affection and imagination also are shamed and silenced out of so many kids' lives. It's no wonder we find ourselves erotically crippled as adults. Why do so many people feel desperately uncomfortable either giving or receiving a warm hug or casual kiss, let alone anything else more nurturing and intimate? Every time someone gives me one of those strange A-frame hugs, I always wonder what the problem is. Why do friends hold their hearts away from each other?

One time I had an affair with a fellow who had the hardest time touching me except in the middle of intercourse. Foreplay, afterglow, cuddling—everything was such a struggle for him. Yet he kept saying he wanted to "learn." I'm impatient, but during the couple of weeks that our affair lasted, I slept several nights with him. In the morning, he started to play absentmindedly with my hair, so softly and gently, with no particular concentration at all. His eyes were closed, and they only flew open when his cocker spaniel leaped up from the other side of the mattress.

"I thought you were Scruffy!" he said and snatched his hand back, as if in some distraught apology.

I never thought I'd say this to a man, but in this context I had to: "I wish you'd treat me like you treat your dog."

He didn't need to learn anything about how to touch someone sweetly. He already knew how, but something in him was terrified of what would happen if he tried it on a real live person. I agree, dogs are much more reliable when it comes to reciprocating affection. But it hurts to see someone think that he doesn't know how to hold hands when it's his fear of betrayal that's really the issue.

Too many people have had their delight and amazement worn right out of them. They hide it, and they squelch it, and they let it come out only in the most tortured little ways, thinking they can control it entirely. But everyone has the inspirations and dreams that can make them the "happiest girl in the whole U.S.A." If you can't remember the last time something pleased you into passion, exclamation, or total silliness, then it's been too long. A lover is someone who can be moved by the smallest things, someone who can touch without fear—who is big enough for the biggest kind of sex that there is.

alone at last

Moral indignation is jealousy with a halo.

H. G. Wells

With a great deal of haughti-ness, our culture declares that the one sexual thing we can all agree upon is *privacy*. The bathroom and the bedroom doors are closed. We say we would rather not be privy to the details. With a knowing air, we say that not only is it uncivilized to pry into sex, but it's also an exercise in self-defeat—that to know it all and say it all is to render sex lifeless. Without mystery, we believe that our sex life will have no life at all.

Just what that "great mystery" is supposed to entail has always been controversial. Is it the uncanniness of seduction, the riddle of sexual taboos, the puzzles of arousal?

I'd say 90 percent of what's supposed to be intriguingly mys-terious is nothing more than superstition. It's irresponsible because the lack of sex education in this country has nothing to do with the pleasure of privacy, and everything to do with being painfully ignorant. No other aspect of public health, except perhaps the nature and ritual of death itself, is so shrouded. It seems that we can't bear to look at the facts of making life, or leaving it. Privacy has been a pathetic excuse for a lot of people's pain and exploitation.

It's not hard to win people over to the health benefits of learning about their bodies. I've got "Mr. Science" on my side. The tricky area of privacy is not the physiological but the psychological, where many adults feel that their romantic lives, fantasy lives, and erotic tastes are not intended for public discussion.

The crux of that intent, unfortunately, is the criminalization of so many erotic discussions. You don't have to actually perform a "homosexual act" to be fired from your job; it can happen simply because you confide your thoughts to the wrong busybody.

I once described an intricate and surreal fantasy of mine, about living in a traveling circus, to a talk show producer who was preparing a program about women's sexual fantasies. She wrote me up on her crib card: "Susie Bright: into bestiality." Yes, that's just how I want to be broadcast to all my friends and family; turn me into the freak of the day. If I had been able to tell my fantasies in my own words, I would not have felt that my privacy was invaded. But when my words were twisted into this producer's tawdry pathology, I did feel like my privacy had been subverted. For me, the end of privacy comes when someone puts *their* words in *my* mouth, when my intimate ideas are twisted for someone else's not-so-intimate agenda.

Privacy is also invoked as a way to keep a public silence about sleeping monsters. Certain topics, no matter how common, become the *peur du jour*, the fear of the day. For example, writers looking for places to publish their erotic short stories nowadays are often warned by their publishers—who put out erotica magazines by the dozen—that no story will be printed that involves minors, including reminiscences of one's own life as a horny teenager. It comes as quite a shock when people who have nostalgic memories of making out in the backseat learn that their memoirs are considered "child pornography" by some legal interpretations.

Where are the allies for sexual speech? The right to free speech, when you get right down to it, is the right to make someone else uncomfortable, to outrage the respectable, and to question everything held dear. Who, after all, needs protection to say they like Mom and apple pie? It's the same with our legal rights to privacy; they allow us to be private about the very things that other people wouldn't always understand or be partial to. We have idealized these concepts in our culture, but we haven't always protected them in our justice system. We have persecuted people (from socialists to separatists, gay liberationists to pot smokers) who made unpopular statements or did unusual things, and the public has screamed when the accused have brought their civil rights attorneys into court. How *dare* they interpret the Constitution for their own philosophical ends!

Every day in the paper I read about another "scandal." Sometimes I get hopeful, like when I read about the woman who successfully defended her right to mow her lawn topless if she felt like it, even though some of her neighbors (none of whom had an easy view of her yard) thought her behavior should be censored. Other times, of course, I despair. Once I helped make a documentary about women's orgasm, and the broadcaster who had commissioned the project was so appalled at one of the orgasms we depicted—I guess she likes her orgasms dry and tidy—that she put a giant purple banner over the woman's vulva when the show reached her climax. When it comes to nude lawn mowing or sex education, the ignorant and fearful won't hesitate to turn to their prejudices, and they won't be easily silenced.

I don't blame people for keeping so many things to themselves—when, in a more respectful atmosphere, they might have shared them. We want to protect our families, our reputations, from being turned into a sideshow or a crime profile. If any of us dares to go public, we have to go public in our own words, because the only protection we have after we come out is finding our allies.

"Well, the problem is with the ones who want to be blatant," some say. My late lesbian aunt, of all people, had a huge chip on her shoulder about drag queens, gay parades, and any sort of "blatant sexual display," as she would call it. But this was the very same aunt who would never wear a dress, even the time I saw my mother cry at the kitchen table and beg her. This is the aunt who thought she was passing for straight in a polyester pantsuit, with an application of lipstick that looked like it had been painstakingly etched on by a kindergartner. When I became aware of gay history, I fantasized that I would call up my Aunt Molly, and we would talk for hours about how things used to be in the forties and fifties when she first came out in the San Francisco gay community. Instead, I thought she was going to chop my head off.

"What is the *point* in talking about any of this?" she said. "You and your blatant carrying-on are going to be the death of us." Well, I was wearing jeans and a T-shirt with bright pink women's symbols on it, but so were a thousand other women on the streets of Berkeley, where my aunt lived at the time. I still think she looked more butch than any of us. I didn't say that, though; I just said I felt that things that hurt would never change if we didn't talk about them. I might as well have sung "Kumbaya" to the Marine Corps. Molly worked herself into such a lather that she left and called my mother—who was completely in the dark about her sister's love life—to complain that I was sending "unwanted homosexual literature" to her home, and threatening her reputation.

What a battle. I felt like driving up in front of her house with a big lavender triangle bus and a bullhorn, yelling, "Come out, come out, wherever you are!"

The year before Molly died, she did come out to my mother. My mom was seventy and my aunt was sixty-eight. My mom loved her so much, and Molly's secret—whatever its point was— had been so painful. Yes, my aunt believed that her privacy, her security, was threatened because of the erotic blabbermouths, the gay rights militants, the militant sex-positive posse. I could never argue her into sympathy or support for all the flamboyant examples—however crass or cheesy—who made it easier for others to share a little of who they are sexually with their family or friends—let alone walk down the street in a parade. Molly was labelled by others "blatant" because of how she looked, and she hated that—she felt like she was just being herself, natural. I was blatant because of what I said out loud; and it's true, I had a lot more control. Was the issue privacy, or was it stereotyping, having your identity defined by others?

As a nation, we've ignored the real carnage of privacy rights and indulged ourselves with the hasty and exploitative preju- dices of intolerant voyeurs. By allowing ourselves to become the Tattletale Nation—we're taping this, right?—we have become obsessed over the trivia of privacy, the mechanical details of erotic disclosure. But where is our genuine regard for an individual's own definition? Even sympathetic critics have asked me if it hasn't ruined my sex life to have talked about myself so publicly. They picture me as a hollow shell, with all my sex life scooped out and baked for commercial consumption. But no, choosing to tell my own story to my own audience has never ruined anything for me. It's only when my words have been usurped by others that I have felt the rub of my pants being pulled down.

talking about it

So many people say they don't like "talking" about sex. They find it clichéd, insulting, insensitive. I am sympathetic despite the fact that I have talked about sex loudly and often. There are two big problems with sex talk: the vocabulary is lousy, and the sex is often ambivalent.

So let's start with our impoverished dictionary. We have a small pile of sex words that offend somebody or other, even though they're as old as English itself and convey some really pertinent meanings. We have segregated sets of sex words—the ones you can say to children, the ones for ladies, the ones for old folks, the ones for the upper classes, the ones for criminals—God forbid you try to speak your mind to a mixed group. Our language for sex—the medicalized, the four lettered, and the romanticized wordage—is symptomatic of our apprehensions about sex.

Take a good old-fashioned Anglo-Saxon word like *fuck*, for example. In our current movie ratings system, if you use *fuck* as a swear word, to express anger or outrage, you can still advertise the picture to minors. But if you use *fuck* to mean actually having sex, then the film isn't fit for younger viewers and must be rated for more mature consideration. Middle-class values are, more than anything, concerned with appearances, and fucking isn't an "appearance," it's the actual deed. We're primed to use our sex words for hostility but squeamish to use them for warmth or sex.

Fuck got a new lease on public life in the sixties, along with the rest of our underground language for the body. *Fuck* embraced free love and repudiated the war in Vietnam all at the same moment. We usually describe the modern sexual revolution of the era as a feat of birth control pills, but it was just as much a revolution in sexual speech. Baby boomer artists wanted to speak their minds with an entire public vocabulary at their disposal. Some were martyrs, like Lenny Bruce; others were censored and demoralized beyond recognition. But in the end, the state lost. The words were free, at least to adult men. Feminism—the wilder side of it anyway—also couldn't wait to use all those unladylike words. "Reclaiming language" came into vogue, to take the richness and boldness of words like *dyke* and *pussy* and claim them as women's turf, not as men's epithets.

I remember arguing once with a lesbian who told me she couldn't bring herself to say the word *dildo* (let alone try one out). She had thrown women out of her bed who thought otherwise.

"But it's a lesbian word—where do you think it comes from?" I asked her. "Dildos are your Sapphic heritage!" Oh, forget sex *toys*. People are afraid to use sex words because they fear they will be seen as sexual—and their fear is indeed justified. If we keep our lips sealed from sexual speech, the illusion stays intact.

Fuck did become a word that hitherto well-bred women used; it also defined a generation gap. Rock 'n' roll turned it into lyric. But saying the word still says more about your adherence to or rebellion against your social status than it says about your sexuality.

Think about other controversial or sometimes painful aspects of life, and you don't see people so upset about the words we use to describe them. No one says, "I can't abide the word *war*," or rails that "the word *torture* is so cruel on the tongue," or proclaims, "I don't allow anyone to say *taxes* in my home."

We manage to discuss all sorts of horrible, conflicted, and psychologically vexing issues in our public and private lives without choking up and confessing that we just can't use "those words." Even words that insult or stereotype, like *spic* or *nigger*, get more public debate and defense in their context than the "seven words you can't say on television." Sex is the only topic where we blame our language for holding us back. We've tied our tongues but good: almost every expression we come up with bothers someone either because it isn't sensitive enough or because, at the opposite end, it's pure treacle.

The first time I had to be particularly conscious about the sex words I used was when I began a retail sales job at the Good Vibrations store, an education-oriented sex toy shop. Most of my customers were women, or men with a pretty liberal point of view. Liberal or not, they still came into this shop a little worried about how they would be perceived. One couple told me, after they'd calmed down a little, "We sat in the car for an hour outside the store arguing about whether we were going to come in here or not." I'm glad they weren't there the day some snotty little boy ran in the shop and screamed at everyone, "My daddy's got a bigger dick than you!"

Especially in the early days, customers came to Good Vibes because they'd been sent by a shrink or felt they were at the end of their rope about sex. They were so grim. I needed them to trust my judgment and empathy rather quickly.

If I said "penis" in front of them, would they feel like I was a respectable person, someone they could talk with easily? Or would they think they had to be as cautious and veiled with me as with a medical doctor? If, on the other hand I said "cock" or "dick," if I said "hard-on" instead of "erection," would they let down their guard? Or would they think, "Oh, no, it's trailer park trash!" I could win or lose it all because of my vocabulary.

I think I succeeded in my vibrator sales talk right off the bat because I had great word-intuition. If customers started using even the tiniest bit of medical terminology, I'd follow their lead. Some people are so timid they blush at the word *orgasm*, and so I'd say "climax," feeling a bit like one of those racy women's novelists I'd read in junior high. Other people just beamed when I'd say, "Put this vibrator on your clit and you're ready to go"; they wanted sex toys to sound casual, like buying sports equipment.

Despite my frequent success at guessing right, I wish there were a whole lot more words to describe sex, from the bawdy to the subtle. Hawaiians have a whole dictionary of names for how a rainbow appears in the sky. Our English language is not as poetic with the weather, and it's a total failure at sex. Our words are stunted because we are stunted.

Some linguistic pioneers have wanted to forge ahead with new made-up words, but this erotic jabberwocky hasn't really caught on. Language thrives on trends that capture the mainstream of imagination, not just the fringes. Sometimes a popular song or movie will make a funky sex euphemism popular, and you can see how happy everyone is to have this wonderful hot word that captures the essence of something we all want to say. People who learn or speak other languages are always adding foreign sex words to their English lexicon.

A couple years back I read aloud, to a bookstore audience, an erotic story from *Best American Erotica 1997*. It's a story written jointly by lovers, Rose White and Eric Albert. The heroine of the tale enjoys intercourse, but that's not the kind of language she uses:

"She's on her hands and knees now, butt tilted up to get the best of his cock, to get his cock against the sweet spot in her ass. She puts a hand between her legs and starts to play with her pussy. She fingers her clit and he moans, he tells her how tight that makes her ass. She puts her finger in her cunt and feels his cock through the wall of her cunt. She presses against his cock and makes him moan again. . . ."

The story, as you can see, is earthy and frank, and the audience laughed and sweated as I read the whole piece.

At the end, when I opened up for discussion, a man raised his hand, and he was blushing from forehead to collar.

"How come you can say a word like . . ."—he couldn't even utter it—"a word like the word you just used a minute ago, and everyone is fine with it? If I said that to my girlfriend, she'd never forgive me. There's just no way a man can say it."

For a minute, I considered what he might be talking about. "Do you mean *cunt*?"

He nodded, cringing.

"I love saying *cunt*," I said. "It's a woman's place to have one, after all. It's feminist spin control. The reason so many women use it today is because it's one of those great words that all the radical women grabbed and said, 'We're not going to let this word be a curse. It's our body, and we're going to control it.' "

I couldn't help daring him. "Why don't you try it here? Because everyone is so sympathetic, just go ahead and say, 'Susie, you have a beautiful cunt!' "

He couldn't do it. I wonder if he craved the embarrassment. I guess I should have led a chant, a cunt wave.

We do need more words. But we don't even use the ones we have with the kind of style and equal-mindedness of which we're capable. We're afraid that if we let the dangerous words out, sex will be more dangerous, life will be uglier, we won't know what to expect. I personally believe we need the surprise; there's nothing uglier than our present silence and denial. We're choking on our sex names, hiding behind the fine discriminations between this one and that one. If I can say "intercourse" with one breath and "fucking" with another, I have just relieved a small moment of vocabulary bondage. I have a cunt, I also have a clitoris, a pussy, a vagina, a fertile mind—and sometimes I have a rainbow of a feeling that begs for as many names as you can give her.

grading

The difference between pornography
and erotica is packaging.
John Preston

$\mathbf{A}$s long as I have been talking
about sex, there has been a per-
sistent question in every gather-
ing I have attended: "What is the difference between pornography
and erotica?" It's an eternal hot coal that will not be extin-
guished no matter how much sand I shovel on it—and that's my
first impulse with this "non-question." It is, in truth, an anxiety-
driven plea for benediction rather than a genuine inquiry.

The erotic versus pornographic debate will limp along as long
as sexual speech is suspect, and only an elite disclaimer (like the
ones used by many museums nowadays) can open any of it to
public discussion. If we thought of sex as a matter of taste and
individuality, as we do with the foods that we eat, we wouldn't
ask stupid questions like, "Is it erotic food or is it pornographic

food?" "Is it the sort of food for men or the sort of food for women?" "Should it be eaten in public or hidden in the cupboard at home?" No, we would say, "Eat! This is what keeps you alive."

I'm exhausted with the argument, and so is everyone else. I don't want to discuss porn versus erotica anymore. I want to say, "Oh, dear, I'm sorry, we covered that last year. It was announced on a loudspeaker during a national air-raid drill last August, and if you were absent, you'll have to look it up yourself at the library." I intentionally want to stymie any further investigation into this hoax of a dispute because anyone who does dare to answer it with authority is thwarting any genuine progress in sexual expression. The very debate itself is reactionary, and it needs to have its pious little robes ripped off.

Here's what people *want* to hear when they ask what the difference is between erotica and porn: "Yes, upon careful examination, experts have decided that *my* fantasies and *my* sexual identity are beautiful, healthy, and a real turn-on besides . . . but that person over there, sitting in the corner, now *their* sexual expression is total rot."

Then, depending on whether you like the buzz of the word *porn* or the insinuations of *erotica*, you pin the beneficial label on yourself and the icky label on the other person. Voilà, another perfect discriminating pose is accomplished!

What's really rotten is creating such a misleading discrimination to begin with. The truth of the matter is that your sexual speech is no better, more attractive, or healthier than anyone else's. The smartest thing to say to yourself when you encounter a style of sexuality unknown to you—which may be frightening, offensive, or unimaginable—is to whisper a variation on this theme: "Let them who are without desire cast the first stone."

The Chart

PORN	EROTICA
boys	girls
hard	soft
illegal	over the counter
cheap	lavish
underwear drawer	museum
grabbing you by the balls	tickling the finer sensibilities
visceral	ethereal
pop culture	Victorian
baseball cap logos	library shelf titles
blatant	discreet
gluttonous	modest
orgasmic	titillating
politically incorrect	defensible
Gen X and raincoaters	boomers and dilettantes

I once had a student who joined an erotica class I was teaching in spite of her apprehension that I would demand her to embrace my radical sexual philosophy. She was particularly appalled by the idea of sexual sadomasochism, which she identified as pornographic. She felt like the only explanation for it would be an abusive and unloving childhood. The idea that it could simply be a matter of erotic taste seemed unbelievable, and rather callous to her.

We debated this a good deal in class, and I pointed out how this kind of judgment—the pathological explanation—has been used with other kinds of sexual preferences over the years, most notoriously with homosexuality. The kindest thing that was ever said about being queer, before the 1970s, was that homosexuals had faced tragic abuse and neglect in their families and that it had distorted them for life. It was impossible to believe that such sexual desire could be either healthy or sincere.

Nowadays I meet plenty of gay people who feel the similar prejudices about heterosexuals; they find the idea of true heterosexuality to be preposterous, and believe that "straightness" could only be the product of a damaged mind. It just goes to show that everyone, whatever their erotic taste, is quick to deny that someone else's attractions could be legitimate.

That's the other bogus quality to debates about porn or erotica—they are often settled by someone's heightened and alarmed imagination about what people on the other side of the fence are doing. People who cringe at the idea of pornography have a much more inflamed and dangerous idea of it than the actual article could ever live up to. Then you have those who disdain erotica, and think it's the weakest sort of slop for the chronically immature. They would be surprised to see how vivid and contentious things can get in the world of what gets labeled "erotica." The conflicting glossary of what porn and erotica are supposed to stand for illustrates what keeps them in such polarized positions.

Pornography is first and foremost associated with the male, and erotica with the female. It reminds me of those ridiculous deodorants that are advertised as one strong style for he-men and one delicate spray for the ladies. Look at the ingredients, and you'll see they're exactly the same stuff.

The gender clues slip very neatly into class differences. Pornography is supposed to be coarser, ruder, the sort of thing you acquire under at least vaguely sleazy circumstances. Erotica is so respectable that it can easily appear in a Christmas mail-order catalog. The word leaps from the lips of that art historian nun on public television, Sister Wendy, who critiques the Great Masters on public television, and lavishes her praise on Renaissance portraits that display luxurious pubic hair.

Ironically, with the aging of the baby boomers, the polarized ice caps of porn and erotica have simply melted into tedium or been compromised by religious fundamentalists. The only people getting beat over the head with the debate anymore are the weak and powerless. In other words, grad students are no longer agonizing over pornography as a precursor to rape, but grade school kids are given a whole list of politically incorrect subjects that they can't express themselves about.

My lover, Jon, teaches art to twelve-year-old boys, and the list he was given by the program administrators of things the boys are forbidden to draw includes subjects as banal as "marijuana leaves" and "nudity," and also the vague lunacy of "anything degrading to women." Maybe someday they'll be old enough to express the world the way they see it—marijuana, nudity, and all—rather than having to follow their protectors' prescriptions for pious living.

I told Jon it was a good thing I wasn't teaching his art class because I might just retaliate out of sheer sarcasm and make a whole installation of vagina-dentate octopi who would graphically display one degraded male figure after another. My gender reversal would technically fit within their censorship criteria!

What has been degraded, in the sense of an idea that has fallen apart because of continual disrespect, is the notion that erotic expression deserves a place in public life—a place that isn't entirely commercial and driven toward the most formulaic common denominator. Thankfully, the younger generation does not consider porn either criminal or pathological. But they are, at the same time, cynical that porn can ever be anything but a "money shot." There isn't a booming alternative erotic industry, because no one is ponying up the big bucks to experiment, and public arts funding has driven sexuality out of the spectrum of public art.

I've interviewed a lot of first-generation porn stars, men and women who are in their fifties now. I was talking to Georgina Spelvin, who made her 1970 debut as the wretched spinster in *The Devil in Miss Jones;* when I asked her how she got from food catering to starring in the picture, she said, "It wasn't the money; that wasn't remarkable. It's hard to explain, but there was a feeling in the air that you could do whatever you wanted."

Nowadays, no one auditions for a standard porn film without having a clear idea of exactly what kind of numbers the producers want to get out of it. What they will be asked to perform will be as stock as Campbell's tomato soup. I think it comes as a shock to many of them that there is a unique personal consequence to what they're doing for a paycheck. That consequence could be uplifting or it could be depressing, but you don't perform for the public without being affected at all—ask any athlete or Hollywood professional. I find myself relieved that the porn business is no longer thought of as satanic, but I'm deeply disappointed by its new hell-is-money reputation, a sort of Marxist spoof on late-stage capitalism.

The first time I ever agreed to let someone shoot a movie of me making love, I did it because my director-friend Cecilia Dougherty was making a video, and she couldn't find a single soul in her Hipper-Than-Thou art school who would take their clothes off and do it.

I was publishing my own erotic 'zine at the time, and she had been very critical of every photograph we printed. "I will do this for you," I told her, "if you will agree that any model who tries to do something erotic on their own terms should be given a medal, just for having the guts." Of course she was so desperate she would have agreed to anything.

Cecilia was making an "art" film; it was never shown on the porn circuit. She didn't give my lover or me any direction at all; she wanted to be a fly on the wall. We didn't rush or pose or move into a well-lit position. When the film had its first showing, I sat in the dark and listened to some people behind me giggle. One woman wondered aloud, "Is she asleep?" just before my orgasm.

I was anonymous and unrecognizable to the other spectators. I went with my best friend, and I whispered to her, "I suppose this should be entirely humiliating, but it's not. This really gets to me." I had never seen myself come, I'd never seen the look on my face, never seen my eyes as I was touching my lover. I wondered if there were any other quiet appreciators in the crowd who weren't so dismissive as the group behind me. I suppose my greatest achievement was that I honestly didn't care if anyone sympathized—I was too self-involved, in a good way. I had done something as a favor that turned out to mean a lot to me, and it's a reflection I'll always treasure. This is the medal you get.

I wish everyone had a picture of their face in ecstasy, in erotic contentment, in bliss, in desire. For themselves, not for an audience. Why don't more people take that picture, or draw it, or write their erotic portrait? We don't have that custom; we've been fearful of it. Even when we intellectually assert our liberal-sex credentials, we hold back because we wonder how our efforts will be labeled. Will we be called pornographers or erotic artists? What would be more dismissive or illustrious? The prizes of propriety and discrimination, of cynicism and apathy, don't look so hot, despite the feverish competition.

the price of titillation

Money creates taste.
Jenny Holzer

Our fascination with grading sex is an unfortunate puritan hangover. But we have another preoccupation that's an even bigger headache, an antierotic migraine case. Need I count it out in small, unmarked bills? Our need to grade everything according to its price—its perceived value on the status marketplace—is, at bottom, our crippling bow to the greater god of all things material and moneyed. Our culture uses sex in the most cynical way to "sell" anything—even though we blanch when sex is presented simply, or sold for itself. The false promise of sex, the illusions we flatter when served on a silver platter, never ceases to boggle my mind. It also makes me want to resist, and that's the first sign of recovery.

Ninety percent of what our media calls sexual entertainment is actually pure titillation—so yummy in the first sniffs and mouthfuls, such a tummy ache later on. *Titillation,* the word, is derived from Latin *titillare,* "to tickle," and there begins its exquisite torture. Titillation makes an art form out of teasing—and teasing is perfectly sweet, but it can never be called satisfying eroticism, because its very nature is to withhold what we dream of and place it permanently out of reach.

It's not that titillation doesn't belong in our path to arousal. On a person-to-person level, it's exciting to dress provocatively, to seduce, to impress, to offer a promise. But the anticipation of actually connecting with someone is what keeps those promises alive, what makes that seduction so enticing.

In real life, we get through those ups and downs, sometimes landing in the embrace we hope for—and sometimes falling on our face. However, in the mainstream world of advertising and entertainment, sex is used strictly as titillation, and the viewer is left holding the bag. Almost everything we see on commercial media is powered by sexual titillation. It's not designed to promote self-enlightenment or human connection, it's made to get you to do something else—buy something, yearn to buy something—which erotically leaves you nowhere. The new car, the new dress, the new breakfast cereal—these ad images are what make up most of the titillating erotic illustrations around us.

It's no wonder so many people accuse advertising and its related promotions with leaving a bad taste in their mouths. The most excruciating examples are criticized for being phony: no awesome babe in an evening gown is going to be my lover if I buy this Cadillac. But in truth, even the more subtle insinuations are just as pathetic. By comparison, even the dopiest pornography delivers more on its sexual promise—the nude pictures that invite you to be aroused for their own sake.

Commercial titillation has the gimmicky personality that fits perfectly with our obsession with making real sexual pleasure either an enigma or a sham. Titillation is the American standard: first offer a peek, then slap the hand that seeks to touch. I'll tease you, then reproach you; I'll build up the big expectation and then laugh at your wish for more. It's that big tit, that winky-blinky bulge in the pants, that substitutes a carnival act for an erotic performance. What, you actually thought we were going to deliver on this choice little thrill? Sucker!

It's not just erotica that's favored when it's dipped in gold and made into a sales pitch—it's every controversial sensation. The free-speech debate in the arts and media over violence and drugs is similar to the argument over sex. Each is a highly emotional issue that has become a tug-of-war over the power and privilege to decide who gets to see what—and how much they'll pay for it.

The greatest censorship we see today doesn't come from moral standard-bearers yearning for simpler times—rather, it's the all-out competition for information, an elite display of privilege and access. The debate isn't anymore about *what* will be banned. Rather, the contest now is about *who* will be allowed to "see all," and who will be kept in the dark. Puritans used to be more old-fashioned, wishing to keep their minds pure and uncluttered. Now they've been replaced by political opportunists, just as greedy as anyone else to get their hands on the information first.

The business of titillation actually operates both high and low, on the one hand with big budgets and industry trophies, and on the other hand in the freak shows and unapologetic tabloids. What holds them together is their notion of the cachet of the forbidden and elusive.

No one actually wants to eliminate all appearances of eroticism. The arguments that rage on are over their aesthetics, the message and the accessibility of the subject to the audience. Those debates aren't stupid to consider, but their meaning has been degraded. Is aesthetics just a matter of how much satin and sheen you put on your product? The packaging may be gilt, but the insides can still be a big bag of hair.

If we were honest with ourselves about our desire to touch and be touched by our most sensitive emotions, we'd put away the high-status perfume, and we'd concentrate on the most basic merits of what's in front of us. I used to have quite earnest debates with people about what they thought was excessive sex in popular culture. I'd try in vain to solicit their artistic alternatives; I'd argue for the opportunities and insist that we need to express our most passionate emotions. But now I hesitate before I ask people if they're willing to discuss erotic possibilities. Sometimes I just feel like reaching for my wallet instead. How much would I have to fork over before the choice of our own bodies and imaginations would seem more appealing than extravagance, phoniness, and exclusivity? People's aesthetics are quickly turned by the color of money. How green is *your* bouquet?

I suppose I'm bitter because I, too, was snookered. I've made the same discriminations, held the same prejudices, and wasted so much time. I was nearly thirty years old before I discovered a world of erotica that I had been afraid of and had felt excluded from without really knowing why. I just obeyed the "No Girls Allowed" sign without reading the fine print. I was afraid to look at anything sexual unless it got a four-star review and was produced by a highly credentialed cast. I never thought about how watching cinema verité and low-budget representations of sex made me feel squeamish; the realness or coarseness of it seemed to make my emotions feel too full, exposed, without any relief. I would read tons of fashion magazines without blinking an eye at the high-toned advertising, but I would be embarrassed by a soft-core men's magazine whose models did not enjoy the buff and polish of haute couture.

I scorned those nudie models for their imperfect complexions and shopping mall outfits not because I was a moral conservative, but because I found them "tasteless." It never occurred to me that my taste was in large part influenced by the most consumer-predatory display. I try to imagine what the world would be like if I'd had the opposite reaction. What if I were red in the face and nauseated by ads for jeans and perfume, and sought comfort instead by admiring pictures of people having sex?

A year ago, a friend of mine who's an editor at a men's porn magazine asked me if I would review a dozen of the year's most popular amateur videos. Jared wrote, "I'm *very* interested in your reaction," with such a mysterious edge that I wondered if some dead body was going to float up on the screen.

"Oh, no, it's nothing like that," Jared said. "It's just that so many of these new videos are expressly antititillation. The actors don't tease to get things going. It's like reality sex. A director like Seymour Butts will film himself as he goes to the fridge to get a Diet Coke, as he answers the phone to argue with his mom, and then in the meantime someone rings the doorbell—and there's the talent, saying, 'Hello! I'm here for sex.'"

Jared's evaluation was correct, and I enjoyed the novelty of amateur porn's nonchalance. The famous Mr. Butts started out with one star, his lover Shane, but then she broke up with him and started her own line of videos, *Shane's World*. Shane's character is a jock who seems happy whether she's careening around in her go-cart or going to a sex toy shop to find enough vibrators to keep a whole slumber party entertained. At the end of her video, she edits in a piece of homemade tape that some fan made of their own Shane-inspired fantasies.

If it weren't for the porn taboo that threatens the high gloss of mainstream culture, Shane and Seymour could be effectively exploited by advertisers right now. Would Seymour be willing to hold his Diet Coke even closer to the camera? Could Shane make sure the logo on her snowboard gets as much attention as the come shot? The true capitalist would find a way.

From the viewpoint of Madison Avenue, it's ironic that the porn nickname for the male on-screen ejaculation is the "money shot." In the nonporn world, the money shot is not one close-up of vicarious satisfaction, but rather the relationship between the object of desire and the object the advertiser wants you to buy. We yearn for completion instead of experiencing completion. We have to pay, pay, pay if we want to join the party, and there's no guarantee that the stakes will ever let up. Do we have the right accessories and brand names to be a sexual success? That is where the present-day sex anxiety lives. It's not about whether we're ready to leave our sex guilt behind but whether we've brought enough cash.

My own work has been antititillation, not by design, but apparently from intuitive rebellion. Even when I worked as a more conventional sex educator, I didn't promote my information and advice as some sort of "hush-hush, on the q.t." sort of spectacle. I didn't want to charge for it. I wanted adult sex education to be available to everyone. I wanted people to be as familiar with the workings of their reproductive and sexual bodies as they would be with washing their hair. "This is your clitoris, not a mystery novel."

I also wanted my audience to appreciate that once they got the basic facts of life out of the way, their erotic lives above the neck would never be banal or formulaic. Sexual creativity is a mystery that will never be solved by commercialism. Our fantasy lives don't know what a status quo is, if we're honest about it. Anyone who subjects their erotic identity to preening for the crowd and to commercial comparisons is going to be turned off faster than they can smooth their hair back.

I look at the people in my life who electrified me sexually, or the situations I found myself in that turned me on, and there's little conformity—just some very splendid chaos. If you made a lineup of all the lovers in my sex history, their looks and their status would tell you nothing about whether they had anything in common or the quality of our romance.

It's not just that I'm without a "type" that I'm always attracted to, it's that I myself am not a type. I'm more than a cashier's total of my various visual symbols. The clothes I choose to wear are pure theater, and superficial glances between each act could peg me as anything from waitress mom to carnal goddess. I am more than the sum of my hairdo. I know, in fact I love, the fact that my sexuality can be inspired by beauty, but I insist that that inspiration fulfills me, rather than suspending me in some insecure notion of my worth.

When I see classic sexpot pictures today, whether it's a *Playboy* playmate or a Parisian supermodel, I see kitsch, and it's almost like looking at a naughty Victorian postcard. I can smile at it because it is a fleeting moment in the time machine of often-contradictory erotic status symbols. The days when I could react to those pictures with genuine envy or yearning are fortunately over. Of course it hurts when I see people who've bought the franchise, who think that great sex is about the right accessories and perfect lighting. These folks have already been pitied or criticized as victims of sexism, racism, looks-ism, and so forth, but that's not what they're really victims of. They are the captive audience of the commercial titillation way of life. If we expressed ourselves, in all our variety, revealing what in our lives truly turns us on, it would make the advertising empire look like one gigantic marshmallow.

A lot of people don't question titillation and the Brand-Name Erotic Blues because they've barely seen anything else. Erotic censorship has become an American fetish, an institution, and a superstition—a faith in material success and excess. I once read a beginner's introduction to the stock market in which the rather philosophical editor said, "A price is nothing but an opinion." I remember agreeing with him in my head and then thinking, "I don't like any of those opinions." I'm sick of opinions that make "dollars and sense" but little else. I'd be depressed about sex, too, if I felt that my erotic future depended on plastic surgery or owning the biggest sport utility vehicle.

How else do we appreciate life? Lovers are famous for repeating that beauty is in the eye of the beholder, and I side with their amorous approach to value: What is meaningful to us is unique to our own desire and cannot be bought or sold by anyone. We may be disillusioned by titillation and depressed by the contest of commercial success, but our erotic senses will never leave us, or be recruited by false gods. The temptation to believe in the pornography of titillation, the smut of advertising, is always going to attract attention, but it's also going to leave us horny and hungry. My greatest ally in my erotic judgment is my constant observation that the aphrodisiac of a price, of a dazzlingly crafted come-on, is a genuine disappointment.

ugly

Pretty is as pretty does.
Old Saying

Every summer I look forward to going on a camping trip; I want to live the whole summer on a riverbank. Just the smell of getting my gear out of the garage puts me in a good mood. This past June, I rummaged around in a sticky cardboard box filled with half-used and abandoned camping supplies until I found the bug-spray bottle labeled "Extra Deep Woods." This is apparently a euphemism for the average backyard in suburbia, where mosquitoes feast in a blood orgy that rivals that of any cool green forest. I dutifully sprayed everything I was wearing, even the top of my head.

"What are you doing?" my eight-year-old daughter asked, peeking around the corner, her face knotted at the strong smell.

"I am now 'invisible to bugs'!" I announced, quoting the copy on the back of the can, with as-advertised belief in my product.

"I can still see you," she said and lingered to stare at me a few more moments as if I might start a slow dissolve.

"You don't have bug eyes," I said, and strode out to the deep dead geranium area of my back deck to test out my new opaque presence.

Something about my little girl's serious consideration of my invisibility inspired me to slip into child-consciousness myself, to imagine myself truly unseen by insect and man alike. I was surprised that the first thing I felt was giddiness, even euphoria. A sentence floated across my mind like a cartoon balloon: *"Never be ugly again."* Funny, I would have thought I'd be euphoric about the invisible ease of assaulting the cookie jar or about all the spying I was going to be able to do, since those were early invisibility fantasies of mine. Instead, I let this phrase float through my mind, relieved that no one could judge me by my looks.

"Ugly" is a pretty serious description. I can't even tell you with a straight face that I am ugly, although I've shouted it in anger and helplessness, and I've felt guilty immediately afterward. I'm tall, clear-skinned, fair, and my toes and fingers are all where they ought to be. What if I were *really* ugly? Then I'd have something to cry about. There now, shut *up.* I shouldn't trifle with ugliness because I just might have to face it someday, and where will my vanity be then?

My vanity is already brainwashed but good. In all my life as a media spectator, I have seen that in those pages and frames, only pretty people seem to convey erotic feelings and desires with any credibility. I know it's not true. I can go to my local beach boardwalk anytime I want, where ordinary people cruise, and I see that sexual attraction is possible in every package. At the boardwalk last summer, the fashion was to wear tight white pants, big hair— or no hair—and tattoos that disappeared down the cleavage. Not everyone was "pretty," but almost everyone was sexy. I could feel the fuck-me in the air. "Everything is beautiful in its own way"— and I find that easier to believe when I'm feeling brave. Bravery and beauty seem to go together.

I've learned that sometimes your sexual feelings alone can make you feel ugly. Your desires may repulse you, intimidate you. Feelings of ugliness make you not want to have sex anymore, not talk about it, not joke about it. Even though I've dissected my feelings of ugly-wrath, and I've cringed at all the ignorance and shame that lay beneath them, I haven't so easily turned them over. At first it seemed easy. The day I decided to reject all the traditional philosophies, religious teachings, and government propaganda, I felt like a shouter, a warrior, clean and ready for my own revolution. I did it, I said that God was Dead, Patriarchy Sucks, and I'd Rather Be Buttfucking. Nuances aside, it was exhilarating to deliver myself from the dominant paradigm.

Yet after writing and shouting so publicly for years, why would I get the "ugly" attacks? Why would I feel shame, when I'd already embraced its opposite so enthusiastically? I don't think it's shame I'm feeling anymore; I think my consciousness raising has been quite effective, if at first unsubtle. It's something besides ugliness, a more constant companion—fear—that gives me this despair. When I say to myself, "You're so ugly," I have to reply, if only in a small whisper, "You're not ugly, you're afraid. "

Somehow saying, "I'm ugly," takes less guts. *Ugly* is small and retreats and doesn't even feel like licking its own wounds because they're too unsightly. When you're ugly, you not only don't want to be looked at, you can hardly stand the sight of others yourself. Ugliness is misanthropy with a wardrobe.

I've wondered how much of a corner femininity has on ugliness and its attendant passivity. When we consider an ugly man, we really have to reach for prominent examples, like Rumpel-stiltskin. Ugliness in men is so extreme as to be pathetic, pitied. Quasimodo was ugly; he was even more self-conscious of his ugliness when he felt the power of his love for the dazzling Esmeralda. In the end, heroism was his beauty treatment.

I don't think most men dwell on ugliness per se, unless they have unusual disabilities or deformities. To think of himself as "ugly" is childish, somehow, for the average guy. When men despair about their looks—whether it's losing hair or getting a belly—their vanity is certainly wounded. But they don't feel emasculated by the lack of a handsome face in the way that women feel their femininity, and thus their sexuality, is on the line with their appearance.

In fact, a man with especially ugly features is sometimes made out to be *more* sexual, more grotesquely lustful, than a man who's more plain. I recently clipped a news article about a chilling kiddie-porn manufacturing circle in Europe, with details to turn your stomach. Yet the strangest detail that stood out in the list of nauseating behavior was that the circle's members were described as "balding," as if this was some kind of clue that they would rape babies. No other physical detail was mentioned. I put the paper down and said, "If there is some kind of anti-defamation league for hair loss, I'd think they'd wanna be all over this."

Too little hair, too much hair, a big nose, a wide mouth, overly muscular, concave-chested—whatever it is, a man's physical characteristics are used against him only as a sign of sexual perversity, not to prove a lack of sexual feeling. Many men do fear that their sexual interests will become too well known or publicly displayed. Now *that*, they tell you, would be ugly, an ugly spectacle—not the ugliness of appearance, but a wound to their character.

It may be masculine to be a sexual adventurer, but such a man must avoid the sort of scandal that turns him into a boy-toy, a joke. Women and gay men who have multiple lovers get insulted with the label "promiscuous," whereas the "straight" man who holds his cards close to his vest can be screwing the whole town and nevertheless be thought of as a royal lion. Men hold on to their sexual secrets like Samson with his famous hair, fearful of being stripped of their power or made somehow effeminate by their intense desires. For a proud man to be called a "whore"— that's what's ugly for a man, not his clothes or complexion. He's afraid of being made that small.

In recent years, we've seen the sexual exposé of the century, in the case of President Clinton. Here's a man with a sexual appetite who knew that, to appear strong and statesmanlike, he had to deny his erotic attractions. He had to make them seem little; and when exposed, he had to criticize himself for moral weakness and personal failing. "He was wrong."—that's what the headlines were obliged to say; after all, he had been caught in a lie, and caught in adultery. The American president and his family are supposed to be symbols of monogamy and propriety. Yet under our breath, the sexually experienced among us muttered to ourselves, "He was a *typical* man." We expect kings and presidents to have big egos, appetites, libidos—those are perceived as attractive—but if the king gets sloppy about it, it diminishes his masculine authority. We turn up our noses at the disarray of his affairs. How can he rule the world with sex on his mind? A wiser culture would ask: How can you rule the world without thinking about sex?

In another period of history, a male leader's overt and even shameless lustiness was predictable, even evidence of his powerful status. Look at Henry VIII! But in the neopuritan age of

American sexual illiteracy, we can easily imagine such a man as Hapless Henry feeling ugly, feeling that he would like to erase this stain and everyone connected to it, for the shame with which it covers his career.

There seems to be no chance, in our modern political climate, that Clinton will ever wash his hands of any hypocrisy about his sexuality. That would be brave, it would be beautiful, it would be a page out of Oscar Wilde's rebellious defense; but it never happens in the Ugly Story. Perhaps the president finally decided that lust and adultery are his Achilles' heel; but it is repression and a vicious double standard that have kept his ugly motor running. It is harder for men than women to realize this, because after all—except when they're exposed, which is quite rare—they get the privilege of the double standard.

On the other hand, there are so many ways to casually and fiercely label the ugly femme who offends: the slut, the bitch, the dyke, the hag, the cunt—she who openly desires, and she who is undesirable. Women—and the minority of men who identify with them—spend a lot of time wishing they were invisible, that their sex was invisible, because their burden of worthiness is so impossible. They want to be desirable yet innocent, fertile yet unaware—to inspire yet to submit. For the feminine-inclined, the ugly game *is* the double standard. The femme needs beauty to be valued as a woman, but if she succeeds as a beauty, then everything else about her is diminished. Of course, her looks must fade—that's the rule at the beauty fountain. Not only can't the girl help it, but ultimately she can't win; she can only be degraded to a lower rung. She certainly can't switch sides without facing the "dyke" accusation, that she's abandoned her feminine roots.

A woman can't escape the Beauty Trip without being reminded that, for most of the society around her, she's never going to be let off the hook. As John Berger wrote in *Ways of Seeing:* "Men look at women. Women watch themselves being looked at."

I'm relieved and thankful to have personally gotten a divorce from the cult of self-surveillance, but that doesn't mean that I'm not vulnerable. The well-meaning lady at the corner store will greet me, "My, it looks like you've lost some weight lately," as if that were a compliment instead of a fierce reminder of what I should be anxious about.

I'll leave her store thinking, "I never knew she thought I was *over*weight in the first place." Then I'll angrily rebuke myself, "I don't care what she thinks," at the same time wondering what kind of zinger reply I could make to her girl-talk appraisals so that she'll think twice about how to give another woman a compliment. I'm a little afraid of provoking her, though. I think about how she must scrutinize her own body, which is older than mine, or that of her daughter, who is ten years younger than I. I'm sure we all come up short compared to the cover girls on the magazines she sees every day. If she knew those models in person, she'd find out just how tenuous their own hold is on the perfect body, let alone the perfect self-image. What a tense little circle of fear!

For all the jokes that have been made about split-off movements like the notorious "lesbian separatist commune," what female daydreamer hasn't for at least a minute thought it sounded like heaven? A place where you wouldn't care what you looked like, where power grew with age, where wanting sex or not wanting it followed your own physical and creative cycles, instead of the demands of obligation and making an impression.

I remember in the 1970s driving down a dirt road en route to my first visit to a separatist commune, where one of my best friends from high school had joined a whole group of women living off their land. I idled the car for a minute before I reached the main house so I could apply some hot magenta lipstick. With *Cherries in the Snow* by Revlon all over my mouth, I'd quickly figure out who was a doctrinaire zealot, and who had a sense of humor and some appreciation for the color pink. After all, I didn't want to escape from one beauty orthodoxy to another one with the same rules turned inside out. The point was never rejecting beauty or pleasure; the point was rejecting our fear of ugliness.

Men and women both fall short in the battle of sexual self-respect, because the courage it requires exacts a price—a price that, realistically, is hard to afford if you look it right in the eye. If we don't have our ugly tradition of fear to hang on to, what are we going to put in its place? Even the folks who ran away to the woods to make their own Shangri-la found themselves still fighting over the same question of what makes a person worthy, desirable, or preferable.

From the view at the pinnacle of ugliness, it seems that equality is impossible, that it would tear us apart to change. I know I'm terrified when I take stock of my role models who have disappeared into obscurity, lost their reputations, or been punished because they wouldn't wear the yoke and chain of proper appearances.

So if sexual honesty is impossible from the Peak of Ugly Perceptions, then maybe we have to climb another mountain entirely. If status-clutching, pretty-power politics seems all that is possible now, then there is only one miraculous route for the radical erotic manifesto: a complete transformation! Let's do a before-and-after culture makeover like they've never seen before.

I have never fallen to the ground to "believe in miracles," as TV preacher Kathryn Kuhlman used to implore her audiences, so I have to laugh at myself for even using this description. It's just that things don't always happen as you predict, or even because you strive for them to be so. Rather, change comes from the accumulated dreams and yearnings of the many who break out of the mold—not because they think they should, but because they can't help it. We become visible because our parade is just too damn obvious to avoid, because fear is simply in the way, and we're too big to go around it anymore. We become desirable as soon as we put away the ugly stick—and then we find real beauty, waiting for us, without complaint.

women and children worst

> Both women and men are bisexual in the
> psychological sense; I shall conclude that you
> have decided in your own minds to make
> "active" coincide with "masculine" and "passive"
> with "feminine." But I advise you against it.
>
> Sigmund Freud

One dry spring weekend I cajoled my daughter away from her Saturday TV cartoons, and we walked downtown to check out a city-sponsored art, jazz, and wine-tasting fair. Root beer floats were promised as well. It sounded like an event we could both enjoy, and it's hard to go wrong with decent music played outside on a sunny day. I wondered what kind of art we would see.

A half hour later I knew. As we browsed among the booths, I could see that almost every one featured winsome fawn and baby seal portraits, droll crocodile dishware sculptures with Disney

grins, and refrigerator magnets of Kewpie babies with their diapers flirtatiously drooping. In the nonbaby, nonanimal category,
there were huge sunset and waterfall posters—sometimes with a
silhouetted couple in the foreground, clasped in a prayerful
embrace, or with a little gilt text that read "Our Love Is Precious." There were an infinite number of teddy bears in different cunning outfits. Beanie-acs were out in full force. I thought I
was going to puke.

My daughter thought differently: "This is the best art show in
the whole world!" she said triumphantly, gasping at one cutesy-
pootsy artifact after another. Even though it was on the tip of my
tongue to share my complete and vicious opposition to her
enthusiasm, I had to stop myself and think, "You know, when I
was eight, I would have thought this was the most wonderful stuff
in the world, too." My taste changed dramatically as I grew up,
and it's more than likely that hers will, too.

What's so strange is that there is actually little social incentive for a girl's taste to mature as she grows up, and this art fair
was mighty evidence of it. When the newspaper advertised it as a
family event, I realized this meant that it was aimed at women
and children and that its appeal to both groups was determined
to be virtually identical. No "real man" is supposed to chortle
with joy and make kissy faces at tiny animal figurines, let alone
clasp a furry baby animal doll to his chest. That's for girls, big
and small, and for baby boys who don't know better yet. The
ever-ageless girl is encouraged to show her partiality to the soft,
the innocent, the helpless, the virginal. Her call to action is a
teary violin crescendo, a flutter of doves, and an infant's sigh.
That's what little women are made of.

Young men, on the other hand, right from the get-go, are
shown the appeal of the crash and boom; they can play games of

death and glorious torture as opposed to attending to Baby Betsie Wetsie. Since they're boys, this can look like a bunch of wild creatures screaming and blowing things up. Nevertheless, they get the glee of the shadow side, the thrill of the risk takers, the romance of the antiheroes.

What they are denied, in the most conventional households, are the treasures of nurturing and adoration. When my friend Cary was eight, he made a little bed for his GI Joe to sleep next to him, and he cared for him when he had a "fever." His parents caught him in this act of love and threw his beloved Joe in the trash.

People ask me all the time if there's a difference between men's and women's erotic expression, and I have to say: Go back and open your toy chest. Look at your photo albums. Ever since you've been playing pretend, you have been creating your future erotic landscapes. And you can easily see for yourself whether you were an early gender traitor, a perfect little role model, or someone who changed dramatically over time.

I was one of the latter. I loved my Barbie like no one ever loved before, and then I forgot all about her. The next time I picked Barbie up I was twenty-four, and I was in the company of some of my subversive friends who wanted to destroy Barbie's reputation by posing her in a satiric erotic photo spread for our self-published magazine. I thought we might draw some pubic hair on Barbie's hard body, or maybe add a clit ring to her plastic nongenitals.

My photographer friends decided not to put a mark on her lovely body, but they did deploy her flexible figure in all sorts of shocking positions, a kind of "Barbie Is My Lover" tableau. "Going Down on Barbie"—it was just a matter of time. Days after our new issue hit the bookstores, a stranger who recognized me walking down San Francisco's Castro Street grabbed my arm and told me that he loved the Dirty Barbie pictures so much he had photocopied the pages for stationery.

Ah well. I had loved my little baby-doll, baby-girl day-dreams as a child, but there came a time when I was sickened by them. There was also a time when I decided to revive and rein-terpret some of the old props. What's nauseating about so many depictions of "women's erotica," and the "feminine touch" in sexuality is that, at their core, they are nothing more than childish melodrama. Just like we play Barbie, girls talk the baby talk; we prance around on little Barbie feet. We open our peep-ers real wide and squeal when anything exciting happens, espe-cially if Prince Charming is on the horizon. When someone hurts us, we cry and cry and cry, until someone picks us up and makes it all better.

Babies want love, not sex, and that's what nice girls want, too. A nice girl can't be concerned with orgasm, because that would make something go crash and boom—right inside her porcelain figure! A nice girl wouldn't want to look at explicit pictures of sex, because that's too vivid and visceral for a baby doll. A nice girl can't say naughty words, because that makes people upset, and it's so embarrassing.

What does this have to do with her erotic life? Well, as I've said on many sour occasions, a woman dieting is a woman not having orgasms. A woman gnashing her teeth over her plastic surgery and her thankless children is a woman who is prompted to use Prozac instead of Pussy Power. A woman with a closet full of shoes and dresses that she can't wear anymore, even though the debt is still sitting on her credit card, is a woman who didn't make an investment in her erotic potential. A woman who feels like a used-up whore is someone who never treated her own sex-ual satisfaction as a virtue.

The most curious breakthrough of my career editing middle-class-looking books of erotic literature—the women-authored *Herotica* series, and *The Best American Erotica* annual—was that they attracted so many women readers. Because of the appearance and location of these pretty books, women felt that they could approach the sales counter with them.

The first *Herotica* cover was based on a dream I had in which the title appeared in a hot pink oval-shaped bubble. Round, pink, no illustration of bodies at all. My publisher was not all that impressed with it and gave the next printing a different cover, this time baby blue with labialike silver wisps behind the title. I've always thought that one looked like a tampon box. I'm embarrassed to describe these attempts, but the effect we were clumsily aiming at was something that would symbolize the sensuality of women's genitalia but wouldn't frighten anyone with an outright beaver shot. We also didn't want to put an actual woman on the cover, because we didn't want any single figure or face to define what feminine eroticism was.

The next two *Herotica* collections I edited were printed by a large publisher, Penguin, who was not as nervous as we had been about putting a woman on the cover. The publisher chose illustrations of women from the mannerist artist Tamara de Lempicka—the sort of painter you read about being displayed in Madonna's mansion, breathlessly reported by *Architectural Digest*. Yes, her work is erotic and presents female nudes, but it is undeniably fine art, not cheesecake, fashion, or porn. The female figures shown are attractive, but they have pensive faces, dark hair, serious hips, and modest-sized breasts. No Playmates or Supermodels, in other words. The backgrounds were magenta and violet, the lettering rather delicate and playful.

What's interesting about these designs is that although they are unquestionably "girly," a slim majority of the buyers for these books are men—men buying for their lovers, men hoping that their women friends will give erotica a chance if it's got a feminine or feminist point of view—and also men who just find they like the story and character quality of these collections better than the average erotica in the plain brown wrapper. After all, when *Herotica* began, the male tradition of erotic writing was dead in the water—it had been decades since Henry Miller or D. H. Lawrence—and even the edgier writers of the time were writing about sex only as tragedy and farce, not to arouse. I had thought of *Herotica* as a way to inspire women; but as it turned out, it sparked a renaissance of contemporary erotic literature from all quarters.

With *Best American Erotica*, I finally had men's as well as women's stories in one volume, and I wanted covers that had a little more bite to them. I knew that the days of softly seducing readers into erotica with fleurs-de-lis and Victorian-era figures were way behind us, as was the pedantic use of feminist symbols like pomegranates and seashells. I wanted male and female bodies on the cover this time. I wanted bold titles and a design that implied a little risk. I wanted the audience to understand that this book was ready for anyone, that I would dare you to turn yourself on.

In retrospect, I'm amazed that so many people bought the original *Herotica* when its treacly cover was such a turnoff, but then we were the only choice at the time. Now there is competition from lots of erotic anthologies, and women are not nearly as timid about their erotic reading tastes. Younger readers aren't even aware of all the hand-wringing we went through to present these sexual fantasies to the public. The look of the books now needs to have more erotic confidence.

I've been elated that I've been able to connect with so many eager women readers. Yet at the same time I also sometimes feel like I am a cat celebrating inside a cage of canaries—women who feared so much for their femininity if they crossed the line into Bad Girl territory. They would never have seen these stories, or been provoked by them, if we hadn't presented them with kid gloves and lace. Why does feminine virtue rest on high-maintenance appearances?

This distinction is even more glaring in the adult video business. For years I've supported women directors who make erotic movies where women's pleasure and integrity are up front, unapologetic. A few such videos have come out and have found a small appreciative audience. But that isn't the reason so many more women are watching adult videos. The erotic videos that have achieved critical mass in the couples market, where women make the choices, are the ones that feature beautiful locations, sumptuous interior design, and cover-girl fashion. All the actors are tan, impeccable, ready to go yachting or refresh their caviar. Despite the fact that they get down to it like any other actors in an X-rated movie, their moneyed appearance is the most important signifier to the female audience. It's like a tonic that instantly relaxes.

Why do so many women feel reassured by the icons of *Martha Stewart Living* in the erotica they favor? Because the single most important message women receive about their femininity, to this day, is the *ching-ka-chang* value of their virtue.

That virtue no longer rests on their technical virginity (unless you're the future queen of England), but it is still defined in rather strict terms.

A traditional woman who wants to be a success cannot let her sexual curiosity take her down the status ladder. That could mean avoiding everything from a sleazy magazine to a man who has less status than she does. It also means that she has to portray herself a certain way in public, in her costumed life. Women's magazines—with all their makeup, hair, and clothes—are the ultimate fetish bibles. This is what women are asked to sublimate their libidos for. Obviously it's a struggle sometimes, and the most rebellious or least successful women just give the whole program the boot.

Nevertheless, the very word *pornography* is a class barrier that keeps many women from looking at erotic expression seriously. It's like asking them to strip naked in the street. On the other hand, when they see an "adult" movie that is choked with lavish symbols of conspicuous consumption, it's a revelation, a green light. Whether the glamour models on-screen actually have orgasms is entirely secondary for a woman who feels threatened that she might lose it all if she lets herself be seen as a cheap date.

Until the modern wave of "grown-up" women talking about their sex lives, the conventional wisdom was that women had to be sold romance and love, sugar and shopping, men who can be tamed. But when Erica Jong came along and said she wanted a "zipless fuck," that didn't sound like a little girl. When a group of San Francisco lesbian-feminists put together a collection of S/M erotica called *Coming to Power*, you knew that Barbie had left the building. When I wrote my first grown-up erotic poetry, I knew, romantic as I am, that I was leaving the baby bubble forever. Good-bye Beanie-acs, hello Amazon sex goddesses. Don't let your teddy bear bite you on the way out.

As difficult as it's been for women to make the leap to erotic adulthood, it's been the reverse challenge for men to rescue their boyhood loves from the dumpster and to lavish a little tender loving care on their own romantic visions. There are plenty of men who are turned off by explicit pictures or who've never said a coarse sex word out loud. There are many men who find that an allegory of unreciprocated love and yearning is a thousand times hotter than a gang-bang marathon. These men, if they are heterosexual and want to be seen as such, find that they have to defend these preferences as vigorously as if they were protesting their very malehood.

Our society's attitude toward the vanity of masculinity is so rigid and hysterical that it almost seems that a man has to come out as a homosexual just to have a heart. The Tin Woodsman must obviously be a fag. After all, didn't he only want to love and be loved more than anything else? He's tender, and he wants nothing more than to increase his tenderness. "Off with his penis!" cry the keepers of the Real Man Registry. Stop the kissing and hugging. If he's going to cry, let him rust away.

Men are much more confident and aggressive than women about finding a way to make their sex stuff work; they aren't as likely as women to sacrifice it. But over and over again, they will hang themselves up at the crucifix of the wounded male animal, wondering how much masculine power they have to surrender in order to be themselves. If they're too soft, if they feel too much, will they lose their hard-on? It seems like a silly question, but GI Joe's legacy begs for an answer.

Some men are so guilty and appalled over their past limitations that they think they have to abandon ship altogether, that their hard cock truly is "in the way" of recovering their emotions. The activist-author John Stoltenberg is probably the person who has argued most persuasively that "male supremacy [is] so insidious, so pervasive, such a seemingly permanent component of all our precious lives . . . that [our] erection can be conditioned to it."

In his essay "The Politicization of Pornography" he illustrates:

There's a cartoon, it's from *Penthouse*. A man and woman are in bed. He's on top, fucking her. The caption reads, "I can't come unless you pretend to be unconscious." The joke could as well have taken any number of variations: "I can't get hard unless——I can't fuck unless——I can't feel anything sexual unless——" Then fill in the blanks: "Unless I am possessing you. Unless I am superior to you. Unless I am in control of you. Unless I am humiliating you. Unless I am hurting you. Unless I have broken your will."

Only a few men have spoken out militantly on this subject, but I can see the terror in many men's faces when they think, "Yes, this is the price. If you give up your male vanity and arrogance, there goes the erection, too! I guess I'll just have to settle for being a prick!" Or others may say, "I'm not a monster, I want not only a conscious lover, but an equal"—without wanting to pay much attention to how masculine sexuality got such a brutal, indifferent reputation in the first place.

But men and women don't have to settle for being prisoners in their little gender dormitory. Girls can be women with real adult sexual appetites; men can be love bunnies and still have raging hard-ons. It's true. I've seen them, I've petted them behind the ears, I've shared their contradictions, and I've even swapped a few doll parts. The point isn't to disown the masculine or feminine characters of our erotic identity, but rather to realize we're hardly all of one piece, and we can't claim our whole sexual selves if we insist on male and female segregation of our own feelings.

I didn't get my own "cock consciousness" until I made love to a woman who wanted me inside her. I'd never felt what it was like to take direct initiative with sex, to ask people out, to get rejected, and also to get a few demands made on my own prowess. I don't think I would have even used the word *prowess* before I made love to a woman, because my idea of what was sexually appealing about myself was based on merely being fetching.

I remember a butch date of mine who asked me right up front, "Are you a fuck-me femme?" I laughed; I'd never heard that before, but I had an idea what it meant. "Yeah, that's right," she explained, "those pretty girls who just want to lie back and watch me do everything—I've had it with that."

"I think I'm about a 75 percent fuck-me femme," I said. "Maybe you'll catch me on one of my turnaround quarters."

I *am* pretty girly—but I wouldn't give up my 25 percent of butchness, or whatever it is; if I did, I certainly wouldn't be me, and I'd hardly be human. I wouldn't be sexually satisfied. I'm only sorry I ever had the idea that what I looked like and how I behaved was anything but a perfectly holistic combination of masculine and feminine attributes. I don't have the patience to be stereotyped as a pink or blue marionette anymore, and I'm attracted to people who get the gender-free message.

The best part is watching women younger than me move boundaries with a wave of their hand. When I was in college in 1979, there were a couple of liquor stores close to campus, and one of them, Mr. G's, sold porn magazines. College gals who were down at Mr. G's testing their fake IDs to buy a six-pack were also just getting their first taste of those famous feminist antiporn slide shows that came to our campus and turned it upside down.

I was one of those young women. Before I viewed the *Women Against Violence in Pornography and Media* slide show, I don't think I'd seen a *Hustler* magazine; I'd only flipped through the slick soft-core men's magazines. According to W.A.V.P.M.'s hushed presentation, *Hustler* and a bunch of other low-grade sex mags were pouring women's bodies into meat grinders. Talk about your worst patriarchal fears confirmed!

A bunch of students went down to Mr. G's after they saw the slide show, and demanded that the owner remove this filth immediately. Mr. G told them to fuck off. There's no love lost between town and gown in that city, and this man had never even heard of a feminist critique.

When Mr. G wouldn't budge, he was boycotted. His business suffered immediately, but he was no martyr for pornography— he was just outraged at some underage chicks telling him how to run his business. Finally Mr. G gave in, outraged but submissive. Whatever dirty magazines remained in our college town, you had to be a sleuth to uncover.

Fast-forward twenty years: I now teach a class on sexual representation at the same college I graduated from. I told my students that they might want to go outside the university library to look for examples of contemporary erotica—porn videos, skin magazines, and so forth. The next week, a group of my women students came into class bewildered and insulted. They had been to Mr. G's.

"What's the matter with that guy?" one girl asked. "We just asked him if he carried *Hustler* magazine, that we needed a copy, and he blew up!" "How old is he, anyway?" another one said. "He was screaming, 'You broads are crazy! First you put me out of business for the magazines, then you say you want it back. Are you going to shut me down now if I don't get you a copy tomorrow?'"

Sorry, Mr. G. Women have been a little crazy—but that's what infantile propaganda will do to you.

the sexual revolution cracked up

Sometimes I wonder if what I'm doing is a page out of a stand-up comedian's script. Say, for instance, I take a seat on an airplane for a long cross-country flight. The gentleman next to me is looking for conversation, and, sneaking a peek at my bag of books and laptop computer, he asks what I do for a living. I've rehearsed at home a thousand times the answer I ought to give: "dental hygienist"—but then I really know nothing about dental hygiene. In fact, I am incredibly unequipped to answer questions about any profession except the one that is truly mine: writing.

So the man on the plane will ask me what I write about, and again, I have a perfect opportunity to lie. Surely I could say "motherhood" or " dead Bolsheviks" and be able to carry on a facsimile of a genuine conversation. But some imp in me can't stop myself, I can't wear a beard. I have to tell him, "I write about sex—sex and sexual politics."

It's like a test; which way will they go? Will they choke on their pretzel, ring for the attendant, or tell me they're my biggest fan? Actually, no one has done any of those things, but they have all continued the conversation. One Japanese grad student at Stanford, who was already working full-time in the computer industry, told me in halting English that he was gay. He looked surprised to say the word *gay* out loud, then he told me that he had never told someone this explicitly. Another time, a woman sitting next to me told me that she used to be a nun but that now she was a sex counselor for pregnant teenagers.

But that's not the most common reaction. Usually, I'm sitting next to a man in a suit, and as soon as he hears that I write about sex, he gives me the eye: Am I coming on to him? He cannot imagine why a woman would tell him she was a radical sex writer if she was not implying that she was ready to induct him on the spot. And there I am, having told the man my occupation, without any regard to whether I am attracted to him. I want to make a point that women should be able to start a conversation about sex without having to put a "For Sale" sign on their ass. I want to champion passionate conversations about sex, whether we are about to have sex or not. But are my fine distinctions making any sense at this altitude?

One especially confident man, whom I recall now only by the memory of his snakeskin cowboy boots, interrupted the description of my latest book and said, "Well, do you want to hook up when we reach the ground? I have about an hour." I suppressed a laugh, thinking about the prim undergraduate who was supposed to meet me at the gate and take me to speak at Bryn Mawr forty-five minutes after I landed.

"Actually, I'm getting picked up by someone else," I said—
and he looked at me like, "What the fuck?" He thought I meant
that I was already signed up for a quickie with someone arriving
from another flight. Busy, busy girl!

In the sixties, the first blush of the sexual revolution, there
were a lot of snide jokes about the easy lays that came along with
"liberated chicks." The slick hero of the punch line—a guy, of
course—got laid at some naive sucker's expense, and the naive
sucker is always a woman. She thought she was being liberated,
but she was really just a cheap patsy who lost her virtue. The sexual revolution was a political excuse for idealistic (horny) girls to
rationalize their promiscuity, as well as a dandy line for male
opportunists.

When a woman raises her voice in the name of sexual liberation, she doesn't get labeled a predator, as a man would, but
rather a self-deluded narcissist—so wrapped up in her vibrator cord that she'd trip and fall on her face if she ever tried
to make a connection with anyone else. She's a delusionary
who thinks her orgasm is some sort of beacon of enlightenment—and while she's finding her G-spot, critics will remind
her that people are starving in misery elsewhere, desperate for
fundamental social change and uninterested in bourgeois sexual fulfillment.

This cynicism about the place of sex in our lives rests its
weary, jaded head on some of the oldest prejudices around. We
hear that men and women are utterly "different" sexually, and
that the main motivation in social progress is the quest for a
material upgrade. That may be the traditional wisdom, but it
isn't wise, it's oppressive, and it produces a kind of discourage-
ment that leads straight to apathy's door.

SEX LIE NUMBER ONE:

> Men aren't looking for liberation,
> they're looking to get laid.

Not many people of either sex are actually looking for liberation, at least not until they get to the end of a very weary road of dissatisfaction. That usually takes a decade or two.

Liberation, per se, is not the sort of thing people count as tops on their to-do list, right up there with finding a certain kind of job or partner or new home. Maybe that indicates our lack of concern for our personal growth, but it's certainly not limited to men.

Men are expected to be horny; they are acknowledged as "natural" for wanting to have sex, but that desire is tainted with weakness, as if their fantasies are an Achilles' heel that will betray them when they need their strength the most. The "little head" of the penis will lead the "big head" above the shoulders, and won't we all laugh when we see the results! We grant men sexual feeling as if it were unavoidable, but we make fun of them for what we believe will be their inevitable undoing.

I say, let's give this wish to get laid a decent shake. What is this desire, after all? The wish to feel sexual ecstasy with another person, to feel yourself completely inside another person's body, to feel your own body open and single-minded and wanting? That's a pretty intense experience to yearn for. It deserves respect.

But it's not always like that, you might be thinking. Some people are totally distant when they're having sex; it's just an ego trip, a notch on their belt. And that's true—there are some cold SOBs out there, whipping it out and walking away. What's so poignant about their condition is that even their stunted efforts are a search for a connection—for that fleeting moment when the ego disappears and they feel something bigger and more complete than either of their "heads."

If men can't express that longing to their lovers, openly and without trepidation, it's not because their sexual desire is in the way; it's that little rat cage in their mind that shames them and shuts them up. Yet every time they get laid, there's that opening again, the chance to be intimate.

A man who wants to get laid is a man who wants to stay in the human race. Let's treat that as a positive sign and look more carefully at the nature of his sexual connections.

Often the first erotic bridge that men and women cross is the discovery that someone else wants them—and that always seems like a miracle when they're convinced that they will be forever alone and unloved in the world.

Then when you do get laid, and then it happens again and again and again, the confidence you acquire leads you to some new questions about the value of sex, about a lover's companionship in your life, about your own sense of adventure and mystery in your erotic body.

At that point, we're experiencing sexual liberation, whether it's given that name or not. Some men will start to question all the things a male is "supposed" to do or feel in the three-ring circus of sexual relationships—and no doubt they will find much of it unnecessary and regressive. They don't want to sacrifice their emotions and expressiveness on the altar of compulsory masculinity. These men are on the first platform of sexual revolution: they're not buying the late model of The Omnipotent Man, all polished and ready to go. Refusing to buy into all the blue-label baloney is a sexual revolution right there. I'm happy to meet such a man; he has hope that there's something better out there—and he's right.

SEX LIE NUMBER TWO:

> Nice Girls get tricked by men into
> having sex, when all they really
> want is some loving romance.

Nice Girls want so many things: a devoted husband, wonderful children, a lovely home, a rewarding second career, the admiration of their neighbors, a great appearance, a new car, a fabulous yard, a Hawaiian vacation—I could write down thousands of things that Nice Girls want to have. Nice Girls may indeed be defined by their shopping list. How can it be that nowhere on their impressive list does sexual desire or fulfillment ever make an appearance? Let's face it, we can't shop for intelligence, creativity, or freedom.

The book of Nice Girl Rules and Regulations clearly states that if you show yourself to be lustful or horny or in any way sexually alert, then the nice husband and children and status you've gained for yourself are going to be ripped out of your life like the hair out of your head. "You cannot have it all" is the warning of the feminine mystique. You can be a slave with a lot of pretty charms on your bracelet, or you can be a fallen woman and take your chances.

Of course it doesn't make any sense. You have to have sex to have children, for example, but you're not supposed to be seen as sexual by your children, since Nice Girl Motherhood is modeled on the Blessed Virgin. You have to be creative and ambitious to be noticed in your professional and community life—but if you get creative or ambitious in your bedroom, your virtue is going to be questioned, because being a perfect wife is really incompatible with sexual adventure. Women are asked continuously to deny themselves, as a qualification for their femininity, and they're encouraged to find their reward in men's patronage.

Admirers are always nice, but they're no substitute for the destiny of a woman's own desire.

A lusty woman cannot put up with the double standard, because acting on sexual desire takes some confidence, some initiative—some balls, as it were. If a woman stops herself from sexual initiative because she's too fat, or her children will be horrified, or her neighbors will gossip, then she will never experience her erotic self. She will probably censure and punish any other women she sees trying it—including her own daughters.

Early feminists had some brilliant names for the double standard at which women invariably lose: the Feminine Mystique (Betty Friedan), the Female Eunuch (Germaine Greer), the Woman as Nigger of the World (Yoko Ono). From the earliest days of women's liberation, feminists have protested that it wasn't parity they were seeking with men's sexual power. Women have been degraded endlessly by the mythology of romance, the glory of feminine sacrifice, the perpetual vicarious living—but we're not giving up the old "virtues" just to trade them in for masculine stoicism, pomposity, or arrogance. No, if there's a sex-positive vision for women, it's of a new society where sexual feelings and actions are not feared, repressed, or promoted because of one's gender.

Desire persists in spite of the double standard; Nice Girls sometimes have to throw a fit, and let themselves pursue their orgasmic imagination. That's the glimpse of the new world that we could have if every woman copped to her sexual self-interest.

If a woman tells the truth about her rebellion, she will admit that she doesn't need to be tricked into sex, she wants it for herself. She wants to feel her erotic power, she wants to open that vagina dentata and take a lusty bite out of life. She wants to come so hard it makes the house shake. Her erotic body is so large and powerful that nothing petite or slender could possibly be ascribed to her.

She is the Mother of Desire; she makes life take shape every time she touches herself and says, "This is mine." She no longer lives to please; she is pleased to *live*, and that spirit inspires everyone around her. There's hope for Ms. Nice Girl yet—she just has to start telling the truth.

SEX LIE NUMBER THREE:

> Bad Girls are making asses out of themselves, waving their sex toys and pamphlets in the air— trying to disguise the fact that no man would put up with them in bed, no woman would want to be their friend.

I guess somebody has to come up with this propaganda, because if the truth got out about Bad Girl Land, every man and woman would want to move there.

It's not even propaganda, it's jealousy. When you look at a woman who's been courageous enough to tell the truth about her sexual history, you see someone freed from the burden of lying and secrecy that wears so many women down. When you meet a woman who has sexual confidence, she's not someone to pity or patronize. When you love a woman who has no regrets about her passion, you've got someone who won't find a leash becoming.

So instead, the envious accusations begin. She's "different," so she won't easily find a family or lifelong companionship. It's obvious that loneliness affects us all, and being a Bad Girl doesn't necessarily make one popular. But that's not why a woman rebels in the first place. The Bad Girl will have to find friends, family, and lovers who embrace risk as she does, who think there are family values in freedom and imagination.

One common denunciation of the Bad Girl is that, while she may have her fleshly pleasures and bohemian companions, she has reduced herself to the Persona of a Boy—selfish, childish, impetuous, and not much of an intellectual challenge. She's all snakes and snails and puppy dog tails; and even if that's endearing at times, who could really take it seriously?

In reality, Bad Girls are smart enough to see that, in the gender gap, they were getting the short end of the stick, and they decided not to play nice—no mean feat of mental strength. There are Bad Girls who are academic geniuses and others who are street-smart or nature-wise; but whatever they are, they are not cursed with erotic ignorance.

SEX LIE NUMBER FOUR:

> Poor people, people who are deprived economically and politically, have no pressing interest in sexual politics. Maybe after you gave them some democracy and a decent meal, then you could have the nerve to bring up sex.

This is the political lie that evolved from the lie told at my childhood dinner table: "You must eat this (boiled spinach, boiled asparagus, boiled cabbage) because people in (Name of Devastated Country) are starving." You must do your duty here, because people over *there* can think of nothing else and must suffer every day. If you think of your pleasure, they will suffer even more. God forbid we think about *their* pleasure, as only the most grim needs can be addressed.

This is a comforting illusion for the puritans and blamers. It's quite a denial of the "needs" that are felt by citizens everywhere. Hungry or not, people are sexual, they're alive to their thoughts, they have more to express than a wish for bread. If all the disenfranchised peoples of the world had their own TV shows and Web sites and slick magazines, no doubt sexual issues would make a prominent appearance. Sexuality is not a frill, and it's not a luxury appearance; it's a part of your life whether you're flush or famished, living under dictators or parliamentarians. It has its own unique relationship to history, and it will not shut up.

I spent many years as an activist in political campaigns and causes. To a lot of my friends and family, the issues I was involved with seemed pretty unsexy, to say the least. I was particularly active in American labor unions, from farmworkers to Teamsters to coal miners. Every contract I fought for, every election I contested, every picket line I walked, was ostensibly about economic issues, democracy issues. Most outsiders think those kinds of issues are really wearing—and even tedious for anyone who doesn't have an unusual penchant for class struggle.

Yet I can't remember a meeting I attended, or an after-hours barroom conversation—and we're talking thousands here—where sexuality wasn't exerting its powerful influence. I'm not talking about discreet flirtations and tensions, either. It was blatant.

The unions I worked with, by the nature of their size and diversity, threw together very different people who normally would never deal with each other on an equal level. Different ages, races, genders, and sexual preferences were all thrown into the same pot. We certainly didn't win every battle, but in terms of confronting our personal prejudices, I don't think a moment was lost. Our devotion to endless discussions couldn't help but bring up sexual connections and questions that might otherwise have been politely avoided.

I vividly remember a meeting where we were supposed to be choosing picket captains. Picket captain Joe Slobo said—later he claimed it was a joke—that he could "deal with one dyke on the picket line, but was every faggot in town going to be joining our cause?" At this point, Tom (who everyone thought was so stoic and who wore an American flag on his windbreaker) came out about his gay son, who had already been walking the line for weeks. He could hardly finish his rant, because it seemed like every single person in the room had to get in their two cents' worth. Twenty years later, people who were there can't remember what the fucking contract was about, but we can remember that night when gay liberation raised its head in that dumpy living room in Cleveland.

Discard any stage theories you may have about how the sexual revolution proceeds in people's hearts, minds, and genitals. One of the greatest songs of the American labor movement was inspired by a banner in the huge 1912 walkout of women textile workers in Lawrence, Massachusetts, which said simply, "Bread and Roses." The song, inspired by the heroism of the strikers, emphasized the sentiment of their crusade:

> *As we go marching, marching, in the beauty of the day*
> *A million darkened kitchens, a thousand mill lots gray*
> *Are touched by all the radiance that a sudden sun discloses*
> *Hearts starve as well as bodies, give us bread but give us roses!*

Bread and Roses is indeed where it's at, and those roses are the scent of deepest ecstasy and persuasion.

I honestly meet few people today who seek sexual liberation out of a sense of social conscience, but that was always on the minds of the people who pioneered the fundamentals of free love. That consciousness becomes hard to avoid once you begin even the most self-centered path toward erotic expression. Even if you believe that sexual knowledge and discovery are only your private concerns and have no particular value for the rest of humanity, then ask yourself this:

- How can you accept the scope of your desires without accepting tolerance and empathy?

- How can you embrace the range of your erotic life without becoming dismayed and exasperated with traditional male and female roles?

- How can you demand your right to see and hear, read and write, what you want about sex without having a stake in freedom of speech?

- How can you insist on a reverent place for sex in your life without questioning the priorities of materialism?

chapter eleven

All pleasures contain an element of sadness.

Jonathan Eibeschutz

How do you throw down the gauntlet to a sexual libertine?

You ask them if they've ever considered celibacy—or dared to practice it. If they say no, then it implies that there is some devastating truth that they have yet to discover. If they say yes, and it is clear that they are no longer celibate, then it seems to indicate a lack of moral toughness on their part, that they couldn't cut it. Either way, celibacy ups the ante for the practicing lover, who wonders if there is something in abstention that is greater than all orgasms, more blinding than any passion. Do celibates know something that ordinary people don't?

For starters, the first thing practicing celibates know is that they cannot agree with one another at all. Look at any Internet celibacy Web site. All that juice they took away from their sixth, sexual chakra now revels in its own internal debate over what defines "true" celibacy. Still, the questions they ask themselves seem unavoidable. Does celibacy include all sex? Or just intercourse? Does it include masturbation? What about sexual thoughts? Is celibacy always in relationship to God, and if so, which one? Who has lived the celibate life who could be a role model?

I realize that few people seriously take a vow of celibacy, and even fewer choose celibacy as a nonsecular lifestyle. Still, their choices intrigue and often impress other people, who think, "Well, *I* certainly couldn't give it up, but sometimes I wish I could." Many people have profound regrets about their sexual knowledge; they feel brought down from their ideal. It's tempting, then, to imagine a sex-free life where you could live above it all—above the disillusionment, the obsession, and the hunger.

Finding role models and fellow travelers is difficult indeed. Celibates who promote their path do not readily accept people who fling themselves down at the doorstep and beg to be released from the agony of sexual relationships. Devastated by love? Want relief? You may not even get past the veteran celibate's door. Better that you should wallow in a few Sex and Love Anonymous meetings, where you can begin the twelve steps of confessing that you are "helpless" over your romantic or lustful compulsions.

SLA meetings, as they're called, became very popular in the 1980s, when the Clean and Sober movement began and the AIDS epidemic exploded simultaneously. I attended one meeting in San Francisco in those years, where each man present talked about fucking too much, and each woman present talked about pining too much. Each individual seemed to find his or her sexual behavior to be their unique disease, without any notice of how peculiar it was that they were divided by gender in their obsessions: lustful gratification versus romantic love. They were looking for a way to find some serenity, some calm from their libido storm, a chance to have a different kind of relationship with their lovers and to make amends to those they had trampled over in their bed sheets. No one said it out loud, but I felt like the search for monogamy, not God or celibacy, was their Holy Grail.

You don't have to go to an SLA meeting to find these sentiments. Twelve-step programs and celibacy seekers aside, people simply have so much shame and regret about their desires that they often feel they would be better off feeling nothing at all. Some of my friends have told me they were "taking a break from sex," which seemed to be their code for saying that they'd been humiliated in sex and wanted out of the game. Others told me they were experimenting with redirecting their fantasies. But rather than being a high-minded effort, their celibacy was actually the result of their shame for fantasizing about anyone or anything other than their partner. Finally, there were those who told me they were trying to get rid of all sex in their lives, including masturbation, because they thought that maybe once you purged it out of your system you wouldn't care anymore. All of these lovers were miserable because they felt their sexuality didn't fit the strict description of what a "happy couple" was supposed to feel, the little twins at the top of the cake.

Celibacy purists, by contrast, are not interested in finding wedded bliss. "Celibacy is a freely chosen dynamic state, usually vowed, that involves an honest and sustained attempt to live without direct sexual gratification in order to serve others productively for a spiritual motive," says one celibacy essayist, Richard Sipe.

Celibates seek their own refinement constantly, and they question their own motivations from the start. If you're a hurt little lamb who got roasted in the dating game, dedicated celibates predict you will not last at practicing abstinence. They want you to wipe away your tears and realize that celibacy is not for the rejected and burned out. Rather, it's a prescribed way of life for those who want a closer understanding of spirituality and self-awareness that is not clouded by a genital-oriented fog machine. Celibates want you to see that life without sex is the preferable choice, not the damned choice; and if you can't see the nobility of it all above your own wound-licking, you're morally no better than a nonpracticing whore.

Celibacy is a choice to remove oneself from the demands of the body, much like fasting or voluntary sleep deprivation. You *will* yourself to rise above your body's yearnings and to seek a divine, or at least profound, wisdom in that altered state that you aspire to dwell in. Many people call that state an experience of being closer to God or to the essential truths of life and nature. I'm afraid I still call it an altered state, and like all levels of consciousness, more than one ticket will get you there.

I have never been celibate. Of course that doesn't mean I haven't slept alone. I've just never taken a vow or made a long-term plan to remove myself from my fantasies and refrain from sexual engagement. Yet my experiences of sex in relationships—rejection, infatuation, commitment, disillusion, reawakening—and the substantial time alone in between relationships, dramatically altered my original visions of romance and sexual fulfillment.

My solo fantasy life sustained me: the thoughts that came to me after relationships had passed, how I touched myself alone, and what I wrote in my diaries that no one ever read—these moments became like oracles to me, telling me things that I would never hear from a lover's lips. I've listened and responded to my body, but that is not the same as being a slave to it.

It's *temperance* that is missing in debates about celibacy; we already have quite enough pledges and avowals at both extremes. I found the most revolutionary advertising message of my life in that chocolate bar commercial that says, "Sometimes you feel like a nut, sometimes you don't." What a reassuring and brilliant ideal! But can we take it? We live in a culture that insists that people must either like nuts or detest them—that they are either nuts or normal. The candy bar ideology is far ahead of its time, and I only wish that such a spirit of acceptance would proceed just as fast in the noncandy aspects of life.

One thing that celibates and sex fiends share is a fascination with the temptations of the genital regions. They see the penis and clitoris as everything from magnets to little operatives with minds of their own. They imbue the cock and cunt with power and prestige. But as a sympathetic "sex fiend," I have to say that I see my pussy as powerful not because I find it uncontrollable or the key to my pleasure, but because it is such a strong symbol of creation, of my womanhood, of my pleasure and my unconscious. Still, it is of little use to me unless my mind attends to it.

If I really wanted to stop being sexual, I would have to stop thinking, because it's quite irrelevant what my clit is doing if my brain is still functioning. There is no mileage to be gained by vilifying my genitals as opposed to any other part of my body. As some celibates have discovered, you can have an orgasm without touching anyone at all—but some other noncelibates discovered that same fact through intense yoga training or a good hit of LSD or just sitting in the sunshine one day when all of a sudden, *boom!* Pleasure and creativity are coming at us all the time; it's just a matter of being receptive.

Some celibates are in favor of masturbation, or even take a Tantric approach to celebrating ecstasy and celibacy simultaneously. Their spiritual calling sees celibate chastity as a particular way of being a sexual person, not to be equated with asexuality. But why is the message so insistent that celibacy puts one on a special wire to nirvana? How do they know that promiscuity does not have its own divine level of spiritual communication? The celibates who offend me the most are not the ones who want to erase below the waist, but those who seem to be taking down the antennae.

Some of my favorite celibacy rants are the ones that concern the release from romantic illusions, from living as a prisoner in that peculiar state called "being in love." An anonymous contributor to an Internet celibacy forum writes,

> Whether you are married or celibate, there will be failings, feelings of loneliness, frustration, happiness, at-one-ness, and love. I think our media wrongly pushes the message to couple when not all are meant to or even want to. I wonder if all the consternation about finding a mate comes from too many people trying to pair off for the wrong reasons. . . .

I agree. So many people think that a flush of erotic chemistry with another person is reason to forsake their friends and family, ignore their solo callings, go into escrow with a virtual stranger, and generally make fools of themselves. Disillusionment is inevitable and real. The mythology of romance that we grew up with in childhood is a candy heart waiting to be broken.

However, the fault doesn't lie with the erotic surge but with the role models we have for attending to our new relationships and feelings. It's so special when we find a sexual bond with someone; we yearn for a mighty ritual, and society gives us the old standbys of elopement, marriage, divorce. Some people feel that they're saying good-bye to their individuality when they get married, or that they are undoing one monogamous knot and stringing up another one. Why can't we celebrate and respect the bliss of a new partnership without thinking that something must die in the process? Why does feeling something transformative in our erotic life mean that we are "risking it all"? We need a space and a respect for our erotic inspirations, without the fear that can drive us to annihilate everything and everyone else from our intimate circle.

I can't fashion a lover or a relationship that would "make me happy," because other people can't simply hand us a bowl of cherries. I'm genuinely happy when someone hands me an ice cream cone, I'm happy to hear my favorite song, I'm happy to feel the embrace of someone I adore. But those feelings come and go like butterflies; and if there weren't something at my very core that's filling me up and making me feel independent and alive, those fluttery sensations would be very fragile. I know this, not because I've refrained from sex, but because I've been so sexual. I took another ticket there, albeit a less pious one.

When I was sixteen and first started having sex with other people, I decided to keep a secret coded diary of lovers. I would put down my age, their age, whether I had an orgasm—very important to me at the time, and not something I could count on—and then, the most tricky code of all, whether I was in love with this particular sex partner. The thing was, almost every time I had a new steady partner, which in those days was a matter of weeks or months, I would decide that this particular affair was real love, and I had to change the code to show it was better than the old love. If the previous love had been four hearts, then this one had to be five, then six; then I got rid of hearts altogether because they took up too much room on the page, and I made up some other Super Love Symbol.

I still have that yellow legal pad around somewhere, and I can't even figure out what the love and orgasm notations mean anymore. Even the simple score I had for evaluating my sexual satisfaction became impossible. What if I had intense orgasms but didn't care too much for the lover? Or the reverse, where I adored my partner even though we had the clumsiest, most pathetic physical encounters? Or how about people who turned me on so much that it seemed like they didn't have to do much of anything to make me come? What if I only came by masturbating while thinking about them? Was that better than being with another?

Once I became more confident about touching myself while I was with someone else, the whole reliance on them "making" me come went out the window, and in retrospect looked sort of desperate. Relationships became memorable for other reasons, and the spaces between my affairs became as sexually relevant as the times when I was coupled. Sometimes I'd discover something about my fantasies or my body when I was alone that would amount to a minor revelation. Even the idea that I had explicit sexual fantasies took me about five years to admit to myself. Whoever was next in my erotic destiny, it almost seemed like they couldn't have existed if I hadn't changed so much on my own.

Only one time did I purposefully decide that I wasn't going to have sex anymore; I was definitely a candidate for the roasted lambs at SLA. It was when I moved from Los Angeles to Detroit—to a much more conservative atmosphere, where bisexuality and sexual experimentation were still secretive. Women around me seemed to earn respect only through being married. The unmarried ones suffered incessant gossip, were labeled as sluts, and constantly had their work and opinions undermined. I'm sure I'd been gossiped about by the Goody Two-Shoes back in my Los Angeles high school social scene, but I had been insulated by a pretty large group of other young people who were quite bohemian. I had moved from a community where I wore a "Kiss me, I'm a Commie Dyke" button to a neighborhood where people would diss you all year for wearing your jeans too tight.

I really caved in under the disapproving pressure. My political work was so important to me at the time, it just killed me to think that my ambitions and ideas would be dismissed because of a "bad reputation." I remember lying in bed at night hearing my married, superficially monogamous roommates make love in the adjacent bedrooms; I would just cry out my loneliness and resentment into my pillow.

I knew there was a sexist double standard—I also knew I was lonely—but my knowledge of that didn't help my own position. What was naive was my thinking that if I could be as chaste as Joan of Arc; that I would spare myself the hurt of my sexual maturity; and that I would be treated like a peer by the (male) leaders of our community. It didn't occur to me that they would never take my gender and age seriously—that as long as I was a young woman, they projected their sexual feelings on me, regardless of what I did.

I finally cracked; I found a kindred soul a few doors down the street from where I lived. He was young like me, recently heartbroken like me, and we were both living in inadequately heated apartments. His warmth for me felt so good—both his erotic desire and the piles of blankets that covered us on a very cold January morning.

I don't remember what the sex was like; I don't remember much about his body at all, except our embrace under the covers, our arms around each other like a circle of gratitude. Life had seemed so grim when I appeared at his door; we were both red-eyed. And yet as soon as we started touching, things didn't seem so bad anymore. My mind stopped recycling its list of self-loathing accusations. His dark brown eyes were so comforting to me, my own skin felt soft. I heard birds outside, and I was startled, as if I hadn't heard a birdsong since I left the West Coast. I don't think I had; I'd been songless, and I'd found no beauty anywhere.

My personal vow of no sex didn't seem so noble or fearless anymore; it seemed like my own idea of punishment, a disavowal of my sensuality, and a coward's idea of penance. I knew that I'd probably get my reputation kicked once this news got out. He knew it, too; I think we joked about it. "It'll be worse for you than me," he said, "except my ex, she'll kill me." We started laughing. God, it felt good to laugh at our tormentors, the social watchdogs! What would they do without their bone to chew on? It felt so good to be alive again, to think something new, to welcome my body instead of hating it. I was so grateful for this reminder. There will always be those who will say they've achieved enlightenment and success by fucking no one. There will be even more who will make an altar out of their fear of sex. I'll say, "I went to the mountaintop, too, and I fucked everyone all the way up the trail. The view is still the same at the peak."

sex jag

It used to be that when the call went out for sexual adventure, everyone who came running was curious, horny, and occasionally spoiling for a fight. But anyone who objected to the erotic inspiration of the times risked getting cornered by the sex-positive posse: Are you *still* hung up on sex? Do you think it's a sin? or a nasty necessity of the species? Do you have low self-esteem? Are you phobic, intolerant, superstitious, abused? If only the prudes could hang their sex-negative attitudes out to dry, the radicals thought, they could be frolicking on a higher plane with the rest of us.

Even the advent of AIDS did not dissuade hard-core sexual liberationists. If anything, it was a flight test we were proud to execute. Like those signs along the highway that announce, "No

Credit? No Problem!" we were determined to find a way to make sex meaningful and creative, bare skin or no.

But neither AIDS nor Jesse Helms prepared me for the biggest challenge of my twenty-year career as an erotic advocate: What do you do when the people you've always looked to for inspiration say they just don't care anymore? I think of the women I met in my twenties when I was first getting involved in our newly birthed erotic renaissance. Several of them have defiantly dropped out. "Don't tell anyone, but I get nauseous just thinking about watching one more porn video," says my friend who made a reputation reviewing porn.

Another friend left town when she quit her position as an erotic advocate. "I can't wait to have a dinner table conversation where not a single person mentions sex," she said to me while filling out her change-of-address forms.

These people aren't ignorant, conservative, or shy; they're just plain ol' burned out. But they still have nothing intellectually in common with the sin obsessors; they don't have religious or ethical objections to a full and imaginative sex life. To be publicly sex-positive and yet be so turned off to sex personally makes them feel isolated, and more than a little strange.

"I'm sick of it, I'm bored," old friends say to me. One of my pals who's been on the sex scene for three decades told a lecture audience that the most erotic thing she could think of doing today was sitting under the branches of a big tree, meditating. A few people laughed, some were disappointed or puzzled. But she wasn't kidding.

It's not just jaded porn stars and bathhouse veterans who are on the erotic skids. I see this weariness and cynicism everywhere. Yet when I ask people to be more specific—what exactly are they sick of and bored with?—it gets a little trickier. Are they jaded from too much sexual intimacy? An overload of erotic honesty, a soulful moment that just won't quit?

Of course not. They are hurting from the gross intolerance of our culture's sexual illiteracy, an endless emphasis on material gain and status, and the sheer loneliness of our society's sexual suspicions. It's hard to be different, and hard to ask for more, when there doesn't seem to be much of an alternative. Celibacy is one way to say, "I'm not joining, I'm quitting altogether."

There's chosen celibacy, and then there's the de facto genre—that of the amused and exasperated retiree from the sexual demimonde. These people have no cause, no pledge. They say simply, I am tired of sex, and all things being equal, I'd rather take a nap. I am reminded of a favorite cartoon I saw once on the back cover of an underground comix: a spent couple in ripped nylons and cracked makeup are lying comatose on an unmade bed, surrounded by squeezed-up tubes of love gel, punctured inflatable dolls, rude pornography, and yellowing penis enlargement pumps. "Do you have SEX JAG?" the headline asks the reader, as sincerely as if it were asking about iron-poor blood.

I haven't used all the broken toys and paraphernalia the illustration portrayed (where is my inflatable doll?), but I laughed in demented recognition. That question, "Are you tired of sex?" has been posed to me for as long as I have publicly confessed, debated, and performed erotic material.

The puritanical revenge fantasy is that after the sinners have exhausted every kinky wrinkle and gang-banged themselves into delirium, they will wake up one day, in their free-spinning world of choices, and feel utterly barren, numb as ice, and further from sensual delight than the chastest of virgins. Oh, the libertines will cry their hearts out then! If only they had been happy with the missionary position once a week! If only they had kept their clothes on and their mouths shut, at least they'd now be able to have a modest, if unvolcanic, orgasm. The threat of terminal sex jag is that you will never enjoy an erotic feeling again. You will have used it all up.

As much as I enjoy the joke, I don't agree with the punch line. Being tired of sex implies either fatigue or being fed up; and although those two sensations are no strangers to me, I can't say that my sex life has been the area where I've most felt besieged by ennui or exhaustion. I could say, for example, that I am tired of working all the time. I work way too much, a thousand times more hours than I spend in any sexual or sensual pleasure. Everyone around me agrees that my health, my family, and my social life have suffered. Nobody asks me if I have "work jag," but if they did, I would ask them if there will be a cure in my lifetime.

Well, what about the flesh tone toys, the pleasure-with-a-feather products, the disco ball of sexual consumerism? I've been cynical about the hype surrounding various sex products since *before* I first got a job working in a vibrator store. But I see the same absurd come-ons in every other part of my life, which is ritually assailed by advertising and ideological propaganda. I'm no more sympathetic to a "revolutionary" laundry detergent or a car "that will change your life" than I am to a "miraculous" set of Ben Wa balls. I don't find McDonald's commercials more classy than one for adult videos. I nevertheless love my favorite vibrator the same way I love my favorite books, my record albums, and my bicycle with the white tassels on the handlebars.

No, if you strip off all the capitalist excess and drama from the things everyone wants and needs—whether it be food, trans-portation, clean clothes, or sex—you will find that sexual satisfac-tion is the only fundamental need that people fear you can reach the bottom of. Even with food, which is often treated as a middle-class vice these days, or as an addiction, no prejudice suggests that if you eat too much you will one day never be able to enjoy another morsel. We have a genuine fear of erotic poverty, that there may be only so much sexual expression to go around. If we use it too much, we fear that our supply of satisfaction will run out—that sexual indulgence is a one-way ticket to sex famine.

Why do we think the storehouse is so small? Where does our certainty of deprivation come from? One stereotype comes from attitudes toward those who, for professional reasons, are said to have too much sex—whores, porn stars, the sex workers. Aren't they glassy-eyed, wasted, their bodies little more than a shell for their bank account?

Prostitution has got to be one of the most personal and demanding service jobs there is; and on top of that, it's done under the threat of arrest. I always said I could never be a full-time prostitute, nurse, or shrink—I'm not even a very good waitress. My impatience would never let me keep that smile on my face and the client's needs in front of my own. Of course sex workers get tired of the work, the pressure, the stigma, the lack of respect. But I've never met a pro who developed an aversion to her own fantasies, to her own sense of touch. It's a testament to the power of sexual creativity that even when you professionalize your sexual talents, your own unique erotic responses remain unassailable. I don't think any of my lovers would say, "Oh, yes, bedding Susie Bright is just like reading one of her books, you just follow the bouncing ball." I may have sold a thousand vibrators, but it doesn't mean that I've always had an easy answer for how I wanted to be touched, or that I could explain the power of my orgasm with an on/off button.

I once read and performed, in front of an enthusiastic night-club crowd, a description of a wet dream I had about Vice President Dan Quayle. People expected it to be humorous, knowing the difference between our politics, but I don't think anyone was prepared for just how erotic my dream really was. They screamed, and I almost knocked over my mike stand midway through. The stage manager greeted me when I came offstage to congratulate me with a special caveat: "You just have nothing left to hide, do you?"

I'm not hiding anything that I have intellectual or artistic access to, but does that mean I have no secrets, no surprises, no skin? Of course I do. Not only is my private life not on instant replay to the public, it's not even understandable to me. I wouldn't want it any other way. I prize my unconscious; I'm not trying to do away with it. Dan Quayle Meets Susie Sexpert is just one glimpse on the highway.

Of course, toting around an image that doesn't fit you anymore becomes unbearable. I don't want to wear a rubber dress tonight, I don't want the trappings of tabloid sex symbols. The last time I went to a play party, a guy in a leather harness stopped me in the stairwell to pester me about an unsolicited manuscript he sent me; he was interrupted only by yet another hedonist who wanted to involve me in a frame-by-frame analysis of a porn movie we were both extras in about ten years ago. Who needs the exploitation? It certainly has nothing to do with my inner erotic life. Too many easy assumptions have made me threaten to wear a custom-made T-shirt that simply says, "Bad in Bed."

I haven't had an overload of sex, but I have had too much of the many poisons that circle around erotic repression. The more carefully we look at our fears of sexual gluttony, the more far-fetched they seem. We spend such a small amount of time paying attention to our bodies in a sensual way, particularly after childhood. We've been taught to "keep our hands to ourselves"; we've learned that our naked bodies are flawed, that our desires and curiosities are dangerous. As we grow older, we start to dismiss our first erotic ideas and inspirations as being juvenile or as an embarrassing tier of self-indulgence.

We basically give our erotic identity all the consideration of a three-minute fuck; then we point our fingers at the person who spends a whopping five minutes on their own sexual expression, and we warn them that they're going to use it all up. How much is there to use, anyway? Why don't we ever consider how challenging it might be to uncover the layers of sexuality, once you clear away the plastic wrappers and the parental warning stickers? This is going to take more than five minutes, and we have to have a sensuous faith that our creative well goes as deep as we need to drink.

nurture

If you never write a love letter, if you never speak publicly about your sexual opinions, if you never dress up as a naughty French maid for Halloween, still there is one way that you might unintentionally express your erotic disposition: become a parent. If you find yourself in a parenting role—whether as the actual birth mom or dad, or as teacher, sister, uncle, or baby-sitter—your attitudes about sex, fantasy, privacy, and desire will sink into a child's early impressions deeper than a tattoo.

The conventional thinking about parenthood and sex focuses only on the moment that you tell your kids "the facts of life." It's some monumental "chat" that you have at a key moment in the child's life, or it's something you leave in the hands of your paranoid school board to dispense in their classrooms. It's discussed as a religious issue and an etiquette issue—how to say just the right thing at just the right moment. You implant, almost surgically, the correct values that you want your offspring to absorb. If you have regrets later, it's always about your choice of words or timing: the message that was too late, too early, lost in the puberty shuffle.

Forget it, all of it. The most essential message is the simplest one, and it's something that begins at pregnancy and continues every day of family life. That is the simple acknowledgment that (1) everyone in a family is a sexual being, from the grandparents to toddlers, and that (2) the sexual aspect of each member of the family is to be respected and appreciated.

When I hear people say, "I can never imagine my parents having sex," I wince. If that's the way you feel about them, you're well on your way to becoming that very thing you find so unimaginable—the parent or elder who can't admit their sexuality.

Parents also tell me that they have discovered, to their anguish, that their kids are masturbating, that their kids have even joyfully told them that they have discovered something that makes them "tingly" all over. It ties me in knots when I realize that they think of their kids' masturbation as a threat, a danger. Even if the prejudice that masturbation is sick has died, there are plenty who still find it worrying and unnatural. Why are we still in the dark ages about this?

My most daunting commandment for family sex education is to have the courage to say "I don't know" when your kids ask difficult sex questions instead of falling back on religious superstition or legend. They need to know from their family that sexuality is not black and white, that sometimes you have to search for answers, and that even then it can be frustrating.

My daughter and I were watching TV the other day, and a scene came on where a boy tries to kiss a girl, and she protests, pushing him away. "They always do that," Aretha said. "Why does the girl always push the kisser away?" And I knew what the next question was, because she also sees how that same darn girl ends up kissing that same boy in the end. Now I had my whole little spiel lined up, and I was ready to go about how sexist most movies are, and how women are always played for virgin fools or whorish demons. But Aretha's question was so deep, deeper than my Hollywood critique. What do I want to tell her about being a woman, and about what women want from sex? I realize that I want her to know, right off the bat, that I'm still answering that question for myself.

But put the birds and bees aside for a moment. I know that much of the anxiety we have about addressing our sexual selves in a family comes from being so aware of our incest taboo; it's our fear of being inappropriately close or confessional with our family. We are often unclear about where the boundaries ought to be and on why parents sometimes cross them. Few things sicken us as much as hearing about kids who are abused and molested in their family. For many people, the only way the family relationship feels safe is for it to be sterile.

But families who perpetrate sexual abuse aren't reaping the consequences of having a free and honest sexual environment; tragically, it's quite the opposite. Sex between caretakers and kids is almost always a secret, where brutal shame and the ugliest manipulation are used to rationalize the adult's actions.

For me, it has been essential to question why our incest taboo is so powerful and relevant today. When I was young, of course I read the standard evolutionary discussion of how families must not breed together lest they become genetic misfits. I remember reading histories of mentally retarded monarchs of the past who'd suffered from too much inbreeding; I heard the hillbilly jokes about a whole family of cousins who had six toes.

But our incest taboo is much stronger than simply a species imperative to keep blood relations from having intercourse. We don't excuse it when no pregnancy results. There's a more universal reason why we protect our children, and it's illuminating to think less about how this taboo protects them, and more about how it empowers them.

From the day we begin caring for the children in our lives, we are preparing them to leave. It's the most difficult thing to face— a grand abandonment of our own devising. We bond with our babies, they are totally dependent on us for years, and yet the whole plan is one day to say, "Good-bye." It seems diabolical sometimes; the timing is never right for both sides, and a certain amount of heartbreak is inevitable.

How are kids ever supposed to be free of us, in the best possible way, if on top of everything else, we control their sexual lives? People who have sex with their kids, whatever form that takes, are doing something worse than repulsive or pathological; they are handicapping their charges in the cruelest way.

Sexual intimacy is the most difficult tie of all to break free from. We look at longtime couples who say how hard it is to get over a divorce—how, after so many years together, they find it difficult to see themselves as individuals or to connect with someone new or to feel like there's a future.

How much more difficult is it when the parent you're trying to "break up" with is also your lover? The power inequality is so insurmountable, it's grotesque. For incest survivors, it is psychologically overwhelming to get a "divorce" from this kind of parent and to find their own independent sex life.

Once you see that the parent's challenge is to make independence for the young people in their lives possible and successful, then you can see that the idea is not to keep all sexual discussion or understanding out of a family, but rather to realize independent and unique sexual lives *inside* the family. It means understanding that sexual abuse of children is foremost about control, whether the parent acts as a lover or a gatekeeper. Locking up your daughters is not usually seen on the same level as molesting them, but each intimidation has its own crippling consequences.

Want to see young people having responsible, healthy sex lives? Have a responsible, healthy sex life yourself—and let it be acknowledged by your family and friends. I'm not talking about doing a striptease at the dinner table; I mean a healthy sex life in the most basic sense. Stop lying. Show evidence of your own sexual health, rapport, and integrity.

I see many parents who go to tremendous lengths to convince their children that they don't have a sexual bone in their bodies. They won't be affectionate with their lovers; they won't admire something that strikes them as sexy, or find humor in erotically vulnerable situations. When they have health concerns that affect their sex lives, they are utterly silent on the subject. They either don't have any books or pictures in the house about sex, or they hide them (in places that ultimately will not remain hidden from busybody eight-year-olds). If they are caught by their kids while making out or making love, instead of saying, "Close the door, we want to be alone," they invent some ridiculous fib about what they are up to.

If your worst nightmare is that your kid may ask you, "Why can't I watch?" just tell them the truth—that your private life is not an entertainment program for their behalf. The same thing goes for them; they get to have privacy, too. So many adults are hysterically equating closed doors with sexual misbehavior; they miss the point that sometimes we all want to be alone.

There are good parenting reasons for being honest with your kids about sex, but the benefits to your own life are also immediately obvious, even if they don't immediately sound so noble. Parents who aren't furtively hiding or lying about their sex life are spared the hypocritical humiliations that their children will eventually unearth. They are blessed with the mental health that comes from honestly appreciating their sensuality, the respect that comes from living their lives without vicariously appropriating their children's lives.

Usually, when we hear about a parent with a "sexy" reputation, it's the worst sort of gossip—the irresponsible mother who drops the kids off at a stranger's apartment so she can have an affair or the father who's more interested in conception than any other stage of nurturing. It reflects the conflict we feel as parents: "Why don't I ever get to have any fun?" versus our obligation to put our kids' needs above our own.

I don't think the natural sacrifices we make for the next generation are so impossibly at odds with having an intellectual life, an erotic life, or a community life that doesn't revolve entirely around our offspring. Going out on a date—or having an evening all to yourself to enjoy a book or a friend—is a very different thing from child neglect. If you neglect your creative spirit, your children will reflect that right back to you with lack of respect or empathy for your concerns. In other words, yes, you can give it all up for them, but get ready for a complete lack of gratitude— and after they're on their own you may experience an emptiness that's even worse than the resentment that preceded it.

Lots of parents agree that they should have a private life, a sex life, but they have no idea where to begin. Especially with young couples, the caution begins during pregnancy, where all of a sudden the mommy-to-be, the "baby carrier," becomes part time-bomb, part disability case. She starts getting warnings from baby care books, and maybe even from her doctor, that certain kinds of sex are going to be impossible, dangerous, or just vaguely inappropriate. Of course, they rarely spell these things out; it's that "sex" itself is threatening. When I first had my baby, I got the usual warning about not making love for six weeks after childbirth. But being close with my lover, physically, was one of the first things I wanted to do when I got out of that cold, creepy hospital room.

I realized that by *no sex* the medical authorities meant vaginal intercourse. They were concerned that the opening from my vagina to my uterus would still be dilated, and more vulnerable to an infection from my lover's penis. The warning hid a hundred assumptions: that there is no sex besides vaginal intercourse, that you can't see your os yourself with a speculum to see how you're healing, and, for that matter, that a man can't wear a condom or be gentle. And besides, I'd had a cesarean, so my vagina was completely untraumatized to begin with. Guess what? I didn't follow their stupid rule! Of course I was sore and exhausted and cranky, but being made love to with the greatest tenderness, when I wanted it, was one of the things that kept me going.

Parents of babies and young children feel that their sex life is stolen from them because their spontaneity is sacrificed; the pattern they've built of seducing each other is wrecked, or it's rebuilt only with the most careful stacking of schedules, baby-sitters, and a week without catching yet another one of their kid's many illnesses. Many people feel that they know what all the right steps are to have time alone together, but that parent-hood ruins it for them.

More than one couple has told me that they "pretend" to have sex dates. They agree to this charade for the sake of their therapists or to appease the friends they've complained to in the past. My friend Chris told me that he and his wife are paying eighty dollars a week to go to a therapist, but then they lie to the shrink about having weekly sex dates. In fact, he's having sex with pros on the phone and Internet. And who knows what she's doing; I'm not her confidant. It does prove a point to me, though—you do end up having a sex life, a private life of one sort or another. It's just a question of whether your spouse is part of it or even privy to it.

I think what takes a symbolic beating, post-baby, isn't our sex drive so much as our romantic idealism. Frankly, it's appropriate to revise our expectations, and it needs to happen long before a new member of the family arrives like a tornado. If you like your partner, if you are attracted to him or her, then you need to spend enough time together to express yourself in a number of ways; that's what keeps your interest alive and your connection close. If your collaboration looks the same every day, day after day, then you're going to burn out, whether it's arguing over dirty diapers or doing crossword puzzles.

You also have to face jealousy head-on; your own baby will show you soon enough what that's all about, even if you're still in denial. With kids, your mission is to show them that there's enough love to go around, that when you go away you will come back, and that they need to respect your privacy as well as their own. They will get jealous when they see you paying attention to someone else. When your infant howls or your toddler throws a fit, you'll see just how natural jealousy is—but you'll also see the "natural" wisdom of separating yourself, with love, from those you love.

Where our partners are concerned, it's just as wise to respect their independent interests, their time to be alone, their right to masturbate and fantasize as they wish. Whatever your opinions of open or monogamous marriage, you should be wary of making erotic fidelity the be-all and end-all of genuine loyalty. I know this goes against all the old-fashioned marriage oaths, but how can I keep from pointing out that it's those old-fashioned delusions that so often get us into trouble?

A lot of couples think that they're keeping their spark alive with jealousy, but ultimately it's a killer. Jealousy is not about lust or love; it's about control and possession. I have a loyalty to my partner that resides in what's important to us and what makes us feel cared for and defended; wearing a pretty little leash has nothing to do with it.

I don't believe you can purge jealousy from your soul, but you do have to put it in its place. I get jealous as easily as I feel any of my babyish feelings, and I recognize them for that. Sometimes I'll ask my lover for reassurance, but often I'll tease him or make fun of myself. I'll shout my most paranoid fantasy, because just saying it out loud makes me laugh at its absurdity: "You're leaving me for the Girl Scout Cookie Delivery Bitch!" Being a jealous vixen is very cathartic as long as you declaw before the performance begins.

We don't tell our children that we will never love other children besides them—but we do tell them that they will always have our love. We don't have a report card going on their lovability; they are always in our embrace. We want so much to tell them the truth and simultaneously to protect them from its harshness. We want to cherish them forever, but we want them to make wonderful lives on their own.

There's a compassion for and an acceptance of contradiction in our love for our offspring that would be just as beneficial for

our lovers and dearest friends. When I have raised my ideals for
what I need to be a good nurturer—whether it is patience, acceptance, sensual affection, or imagination—then I have raised my
own quality of life, my passion for everything. Many people have
been proud to say that being a parent made them better people;
but because of our ill-understood taboos, parents have been
afraid to say that their maturity as nurturers made them better
lovers as well.

souled-out sex

Sensuality isn't worth a hair more than spirituality,
and it's the same the other way around. It's all one,
everything is equally good. Whether you embrace a
woman or make a poem, it's the same. So long as
the main thing is there, the love, the burning, the
emotion, it doesn't matter whether you are a monk
on Mount Athos or a man about town in Paris.

Hermann Hesse

Shortly after I began writing this book, I went to see my chiropractor—a woman who's brought me a great deal of pain relief, healing, and body awareness over the years.

When I told her I was writing a new book about creativity and eroticism, she winced and said, "Oh, no, it's not going to be *The Soul of Sex*, is it? I'm so sick of those books with *soul* in the title."

I immediately sympathized with her anxiety. The New Age influence is so pervasive, and its definitions so fuzzy, that faced with anything having to do with spirituality, many people feel only pure dread. There is so much chicanery, and so many Let's-Make-a-Quick-Buck-off-Your-Soul activities in the fields of alternative health and spirit, that even to talk about the soulful aspects of sex seems to invite a hot dose of skepticism—my own in particular.

My first major embarrassment in the New Age Sex Wars happened when I worked at Good Vibrations, which had a very good library of books on every aspect of sexuality. I was eager to have something on hand to suit every customer's dream or dilemma, and I was surprised to see how many men were coming in and asking for a good book on Tantric sex.

I grew up with parents who had lived in India in the 1950s—before the patchouli-incense youth explosion—and my acquaintance with Tantra had to do with the classical books and art I had examined at home. The literature, I knew, was eloquent (albeit rather retrograde in the gender department) on the topic of physical and spiritual fulfillment. Gosh, what a surprise to find so many men taking an interest in Hinduism!

As I spoke to these customers in more detail, however, I realized that few of them had any serious interest in religion, sacred texts, or history. What they thought Tantra meant was "how to get an erection whenever I want one and keep it going for hours and hours without flagging." They were impressed by notions of Hindu gods who are endlessly virile and who have luscious babes in saris falling all over themselves trying to worship their lingam. They thought that Tantra is a physical trick, like wiggling your ears, that will produce the ultimate hard-on. Plus, they were so upset about what they regarded as their inferior sexual performance that they were eager to try any sort of chanting, cock rings, or yoga headstands to achieve mastery over their phallus.

Understanding their true motives made me want to eliminate any book with the word *Tantra* from our shop. These men were being sorely misled about the real nature of sexual satisfaction (not to mention Hinduism)—and about how to change their sexual responses if they wanted to. Those same customers have now abandoned their earnest treks to Indian mysticism and instead are demanding Viagra.

There is only one "secret" to prolonging one's erection before climax, and it is common to every culture and religious background: masturbation. I know the word doesn't have the cachet of the *Kama Sutra*, but the simple fact is that men who experiment and play with their arousal, getting to know every nuance of their genitals and reactions, are the ones who have the most control over their ejaculation.

Women, too, gain the best knowledge of their orgasm through masturbating. Some may fantasize about the perfect lover who has the time and expertise to thoroughly explore and understand their body. But even if such a dream lover existed, it would not be the same as the knowledge gained through self-touch.

Certainly breath control, fantasy, and creative thinking can all influence an orgasm, but at a certain point you have to acknowledge your own body's responses and practice them. It's this kind of "fooling around" that is most effectively done when you're not performing for anyone, when you're alone and can concentrate simply on your own body and thoughts.

Men are accustomed to associating masturbation with juvenile behavior, with the guy who "can't get any." Most married men are regular masturbators, but no doubt many of them are ashamed of that fact or hide it from their partners, as if it were a rejection of their spouse. Masturbation is not a rejection of anyone, and although Tantric philosophy will lead you to similar egoless conclusions, you don't need to take a quick pass at a centuries-old religious practice to get that simple message. When I tell men to save the Tantric chitchat and start jerking off with pride, they can barely believe me. But it's true—every tip, every treatment, every spiritual practice that addresses sexuality has self-discovery through masturbation at its core.

Some people associate masturbation with some sort of selfish isolation—the sure way to never go out on a date again, because you're so infatuated with your own hand. But why do we think that solo erotic practice is so different from, say, violin practice? Do we listen to musicians rehearsing their instrument and bemoan the fact that they're never going to want to play with anyone else ever again? No, our practice as solo lovers gives us some of the most precious knowledge that we can bring to our partners.

Some of my spiritual-seeking customers were offended that I even mentioned their penis in the first place. What they wanted was a sexual ecstasy that built up in their heart and filled their whole body with light—the kind of One-God, One-Love, One-Bliss-Out eroticism that didn't dwell in the lowly genital regions. Many women on the New Age erotic path felt this way as well—that a physical orgasm was only a speck of what sexual enlightenment could really mean.

Part of me was quick to agree with them. I was delighted that they didn't think of their sexual bodies as mere machines that you pump quarters into and pull the handle. I've had great sex without any erections whatsoever; I've had kisses that bordered on extrasensory hallucinations; I know what a look across a crowded room can do to your body temperature. Everything about sexual pleasure is initiated in our minds, and this capacity is legendary.

Yet I also could see a certain judgment against lust and physical gratification from some of the New Age books and teachers. Some of this is because teachings based on various religions (whether Hinduism, Islam, or Judaism) are just as influenced by puritanical, ascetic, and sexist traditions as is Christianity.

It's not that far from being an uptight WASP, shamed about sex and its attendant desires, to being a New Age Seeker who disdains all the earthly appetites. Such people believe that if they lose their need for food, sleep, and sex, they will get closer to God. I think they're getting closer to losing their minds. Their wish to lose their "animal" self, to be closer to enlightenment, ignores the fact that our bodies are not simply ungainly and distracting containers; our creaturehood is essential to our creative powers.

If you are drawn to a nontraditional, non-Western ideology, ask yourself where sexual liberation lies in its philosophy. Are masculine and feminine roles fluid and accommodating, or are they drawn to fit a predetermined role? Does your faith tell you that masturbation is selfish, that it wastes one's precious energy? Or that monogamy is the only mature relationship in the eyes of your God? Are you led to believe that your sexual satisfaction is something that only your faith can give you, or something that must be sacrificed to get closer to essential truths?

If any of these Rules of Living sound familiar, ask yourself why something that is supposed to be so very divine and far-reaching—a tradition far beyond your own conventional church upbringing—would hand you the same load of body-loathing, double-standard, sexually shaming intolerance. Where's the higher ground in that?

I lost two lovers, who I cared for deeply, to the conservative and oppressive wings of alternative religions. It would be easy to call their groups crazy cults—but then I always thought it was unfair to call someone in a turban a cult member while treating a Roman Catholic bishop as if he were perfectly legitimate. A religion is just a cult whose bank account has reached critical mass; witness the sterling success of the Moonies and the Scientologists.

I was curious to see how my converted lovers would treat the sexual concerns that they had before they joined their new church. One of them, my boyfriend Mark, worried that he failed to keep an erection as long as he thought he was supposed to; he ignored the fact that I was satisfied, and he disregarded the pleasure of his own orgasm. It also troubled him when we had any kind of sex that reminded him of homosexuality. I was so naive about what triggers men's "Am a I fag?" hallucinations that I had to pester him to tell me what he was in such a stew about.

Finally, he copped to it: he was ashamed when I played with his ass, even though it gave him intense pleasure. The most revealing thing he ever told me was how, when I was embracing him from behind in the shower, he fantasized that my hands on his cock were really a man's. To my surprise, I found the thought arousing. I hadn't known my touch was so potent. I said, "Why worry about 'being gay' when you like sex with me so much? I don't care if you think about men when we're together. It's me who's touching you! Just give it up!" In hindsight, I should have just pushed him into the shower again without any explanation.

Of course it was easier for me to give advice than for him to cut through the umbilical guilt. When he joined up with a famous Guru X a few years later, long after our affair, I couldn't wait to ask him how his new religion affected his sex life. He very patronizingly gave me a list of strict rules that all the faithful had to abide by. Masturbation was out; that was the top of the list. Guru X didn't want to see any wasted drops. Meanwhile, Mark still had nothing but complaints about his penis. In fact, he insulted himself worse than ever; but now, instead of having someone like me urging him to break loose, he had a big papa figure to furnish all the prohibition and criticism he could swallow.

It was no surprise to me, a few years later, when a whole bunch of women started suing Guru X for rape and sexual harassment, accusing him of breaking every rule he set for his followers. Mark defended him, determined to hold on to Papa's Rules for Clean Living and Sure-Fire Enlightenment, rather than admit that behind every erotic condemnation there's a burning hypocrite.

I wish my old friend would come out of his fantasy closet; I wish he could accept whatever small or large percent of him is bisexual. I wish he would love his penis as part of his pleasure-giving-and-receiving body. I wish he could understand his erotic spirit as a gift to his desire for social transformation instead of something that betrays it.

My next sweetheart who crossed over into a spiritual black hole was a young woman named Mary, who came to my bed while I was crying my eyes out over being dumped by someone else. At first she was a sweet comfort to me, and then I saw that she was seeking something from me as well: she had a one-track sexual longing to give herself up, to push past any kind of resistance into bottomless erotic submission. Well, I should say it appeared bottomless to me then, because I barely knew the first thing about S/M, and I had no idea how I was supposed to handle her.

Mary liked me to fuck her so hard that it would scare me— because of the rush it gave me, as well as my fear that I would hurt her. As is so often the case in sexual dilemmas, the only thing that was "hurting" us was our ignorance. If we'd read a chapter or two from any decent handbook on deep penetration, I'm sure I could have dissolved my guilt and worries on the spot.

One day I called her in the afternoon, and she told me in the strangest sort of monotone to come collect my things. When I asked her what was wrong, she told me she'd had an overnight conversion to join a tribe called Zendyck and that she was leaving in a few hours. I drove up to her cabin with a friend to see her looking like a magenta scarecrow, dying all her clothes pink in a giant vat, with a vicious little rat of a man doing all the talking for her.

Her bank account—liquidated for Mr. Zendyck. Her sexuality—completely under this lunatic's lock and key. I felt like I was in an episode of *The Return of Charlie Manson*. Here I'd been worried about the consequences of tying her up to our headboards, and now she was completely ensnared in this madman's rhetoric.

To her, it wasn't mad. She was leaving to go tend his flock in the desert, to panhandle in the streets for more money, to lose her period from lack of eating, and to follow whatever sexual demands or prohibitions he cooked up for the day. It was Guru as Pimp all over again. A year later, Mr. Zendyck sent her out to sell their "newspaper" for spare change, and for some reason, she made a collect call to my apartment in San Francisco and asked me to wire her a train ticket. She didn't admit she was walking out; she just said she was really tired and she needed to go to sleep for a while.

Brainwashing, along with depriving you of all your basic desires, makes you tired beyond all reason. My friend seemed to be learning how to walk again, and she was mistrustful of every step. When she physically recovered, she moved to the country, and told me she'd met a new love. She called herself a lesbian separatist now. I was a little disappointed but mostly relieved. As New Age experiments go, lesbian separatism is pro-sex, pro-art, propelled by consensus decision making, and fortified by a wholesome vegetarian diet. As an antidote to Zendyck, it sounded perfect.

I think both of my friends' conversions were motivated largely by fear, and one of those core fears was their sense of shame and helplessness over their sexual passion. They wanted a discipline that would silence that imagination and yearning, so they could sublimate—at least partially—their sexual taste for submission with the subordinations of their new faith.

Of course one does not want to be consumed with lust to the destruction of all else, but why is that our first fear? Why do we think that if we let ourselves embrace the power of touch, we will be swept off on a tide of anarchy and disintegration? We are mesmerized by forbidden fruit, and we imagine that the first bite will unhinge us from all our duties and obligations. But any obligation that surrenders a sexual life is an obligation to be questioned.

The truth is that sexual creativity is healthy for your mind, it is comforting and healing to your fatigue, it is an inspiration at times when things feel unbearable. A loss of libido is a sign of depression and/or illness, not an ascension to sainthood or the inevitable bow to practicalities.

So where does one find a love life that combines mind, body, and spirit, with pleasure intact? The sexual revolution in the New Age may have started with massage oils and Tantric gurus (the massage oil is a sounder proposition than the guru), but in its latest incarnation, the positive-sex posse in the New Age is decidedly pagan. Pagan beliefs are strained no more purely than those of any other faith, but they do have a joyful approach to pleasure, a rejection of "sin" as well as of holy patriarchs of any sort. The connotations of paganism have always had a bacchanalian air to them; they make you think of people who are furry and fuckable and in tune with the seasons; they dance and eat and drink their ambrosia.

Why are so many spiritual movements obsessed with eradicating the sexual? Why are they transparently attached to chauvinistic displays toward women, children, and men's own feminine side? The pope, Zendyck, the Promise Keepers, and Guru X ought to all have a big roast so they can ream one another vituperatively. I remember Mark once griping how unfair it was that I dismissed his cult leader just because I disagreed with "one thing"—the prohibition on masturbation. I'm sure I'm the only person he ever met who proposed masturbation as a litmus test. Well, I can't imagine any test more articulate: it fingers the common point among all sex suppressors—that repression of the body is prerequisite to subordination.

chapter fifteen

God, I can push the grass apart
And lay my finger on Thy heart!
Edna St. Vincent Millay

I used to have a relationship with God; I begged him to save my life on a few occasions. I do mean "begged," on my knees and making insane promises—and when the peril passed over, and I was still alive, I thanked him for saving me. I was a child, and there were troubles in my family sometimes that made me think I wasn't going to make it.

My biggest promise to God—now don't laugh—came in the form of a trade with him. If he saved my life, I would become a nun and start a convent in some really deserving location. I remember, as I grew up, that I started having other ambitions for what I'd like to do, and I began to wonder if I could negotiate a time limit on that convent pledge.

What an ungrateful fantasy! The nuns I studied under warned us, again and again, not to treat God like a parachute cord: he wanted our devotion all the time, not just when we were desperate. Their reprimands guilt-tripped me but didn't change my position much. In truth, the only time I was utterly committed to God's existence was when I was begging for rescue. "Save me! I will turn my life over to you if you do." When I decided, in puberty, that I no longer believed in God—and it was an abrupt decision—one of the things I felt a little silly about was that I had cried out for a savior in the first place.

Recently I talked with my lover about his experience being raised as an atheist, compared to my upbringing as an Irish American Catholic. I asked him, "If you were in an airplane going down for a crash, would you feel like praying all of a sudden?" I confessed that in spite of myself, I would probably revert to my childhood begging, because that's my emotional last resort.

"No," he said, "I couldn't, because it's never had any meaning to me. I'd probably be trying to figure out how the flotation cushion works." But then he added, "I don't think you should be ashamed of wanting to be rescued; someone should have saved you when you were helpless as a kid, and it should have been a flesh-and-blood someone."

My release from God happened as an adolescent, when I was becoming more powerful, more independent, and certainly more sexual. I moved from one parent's home to the other. My father, whom I was getting to know for the first time, told me he was a Zen Buddhist and had been since the fifties. My new friends in high school told me they were Marxists. The girls I baby-sat with in my neighborhood told me that yeah, God exists, but she is only discovered after chewing a lot of peyote. I revived my own interest in myth and religious traditions, not because I was a seeker, but because I just couldn't resist a good story.

The last straw came when I was invited to some sort of Jewish Unitarian service, where the word *God* never came up. The service took place in a basement with no stained glass, flowers, candles, or statues. These people had no concept of God saving their ass; they were all community activists. I walked out that night and directly addressed the stars: "You don't exist, do you? That means I don't have to join a convent! If I'm wrong, and you really are up there, then I hope you're not too disappointed. There's got to be more than one way to make a sacrifice."

It occurs to me now that it's odd I didn't have an equally earnest conversation with the Devil, since in childhood I had addressed him so many more times than Jesus. I had personally asked the Devil over and over again to leave me alone. At one point, in my campaign to stop masturbating—this was the place where I really felt the Devil and I were closest—I just said, "Okay, I give up, you win. Burn me away." As sketchy as my Catholic education had been on the whys and wherefores of heaven and enlightenment, I had the whole manual on hell.

Nowadays, although I am open to many people's conceptions of God and divinity, I have zero tolerance for devilmongering. I've tried very hard to let my own daughter see that there are a lot of spiritual traditions to learn from, and I don't make fun of her desire to believe in something outside of our material conditions. But the day she came home in tears telling me that some girls in class told her she would "go to hell" if she didn't believe in Jesus Christ, I blew up. "That's crap," I said—the first unequivocal opinion I'd shared with her on religion. "There is no such thing as hell; they're just trying to bully you."

What are little girls told about Hell and the Devil? The Devil is the one who tempts you; and temptation is almost always manifested as (a) mouthing off and being sassy, (b) being angry and unremorseful, and (c) feeling sexual pleasure.

When a young woman discovers her power, both sexual and intellectual, she unleashes her own voice, her righteousness. The first things she has to jettison are the Devil and any religious representation of her gender as stained or subservient. She's just naturally going to be attracted to Goddesses or witches or, as in my case, a scientific understanding of the body and a historical view of sexual politics.

I've always hesitated to call myself an atheist or agnostic, because religious labels, like sex labels, change endlessly in sectarian debates. Instead, I find faith in the fact that almost anything is possible and that virtually nothing is certain. It's easy for me to believe that there's something bigger than we are, because I don't think our species is that brilliant. Look at how often we find ourselves staring at the simplest things in the universe with awe. Our most truthful answer to the biggest questions is often "I don't know." I'm convinced of our modest place in the universe.

The closest I get to spiritual essence is when I feel unencumbered by my everyday consciousness, and that happens most vividly in dreams, in artistic inspiration, in erotic life, and in love. I know that I'll look back on some of those experiences as flights of fancy, especially overwrought personal indulgences. But even in its most childish and irrational expression, where did that ball of fire come from? It can't all be an undigested bit of beef.

I also savor the idea of the temple communion, the gathering of the beloved. Even though my conventional church experiences were nothing but a tedious spell of alienation, I found my own communion when I became a political animal. In demonstration, vigil, sit-in, and pie fight, I felt the power of turning an unfair battle upside down, the steadfastness of the dearest comrades, the love of a vision. That vision may have crumbled at several points, but the bonds of our community persisted.

The first time I ever went to something that could be called an orgy, I found another community. I was knocked out by the combination of sex and group ritual. Here, sexual connection was undisguised, but it was bigger than one couple, so that instead of some little blazing romance between A and B, you had the bonfire of critical mass. The feeling of sexual arousal, which always makes me feel bigger than myself, complemented the experience of loving a community, where knowing names is not as important as an unforgettable group experience.

(I don't mean to give the impression that every sex party is nirvana. I can't even claim that I've had the best sex of my life at an orgy; I've been to some real duds, where groups of stick-in-the-muds stood around empty beds discussing their corns and their tax exemptions.)

I've had some of my best "consciousness" experiences at play parties, because I was so aware of how shocking it was—the classic "delightfully shocking"—to have friendship and sexuality and collaboration outside the rules of paired and possessive living. I like any group that calls for a reassessment of my assumptions.

It's hard for me to restrain my boosterism about sexual experimentation, whether it's having sex with more than one person or writing an erotic fantasy down, or making love to yourself outside. Really, the actions are subordinate to the idea that sex can be different from what you've been raised to believe. It can be self-knowledge—inspiring, communicative, metaphysical—instead of

just the old in-and-out, the pink-and-blue uniforms, dutiful or
dirty.

It annoys me to be labeled an acolyte or a minister of sexual
excess. Sexual creativity is not a religion; it neither gives you a
seat next to serenity nor drives you away. Unbridled eroticism
will not solve your problems, not because sex isn't healing, but
because there are no magic bullets. Sex is more like the magic
question—the question you want to spend a lifetime answering.
I never feel like shaking a finger: "It would be good for you if you
did this. . . . You would be a better person if only . . ." That kind
of instruction makes me cringe. Plenty of know-nothings out
there have colorful sex lives, if one is simply counting orgasms,
locations, or outfits.

But the notion that sexual power is intelligence, that sexual
respect should be a part of any decent philosophy, that erotic
tolerance is a sign of civilization rather than decadence—that is
the higher ground. There's a reason that the community spirit of
sexual liberation has always been communalistic and commu-
nistic. It's one thing to maintain an isolated conceit about your
own little kink, but when groups of like-minded "deviants"
come together to talk, they find that their philosophical discussions lead them to ethical issues about consent, integrity, fair-
ness. Sexual freedom movements have never been led by bigots
or hawks or isolationists.

Why, then, are there groups of gay Republicans and libertine fiscal conservatives? Because, honestly, those people's
identities have been formed in discussing sexual civil
rights rather than sexual liberation. If they talked more about
their sexuality, they might have a harder time placing their
first priority on the economic bottom line. Like spirituality,
sexual transformation raises issues of empathy, compassion,

and humility, and these undermine the notion that survival demands a me-first credo.

Believing in the beneficial power of sexual imagination is not bowing down to a new god, giving up your feeble protests to Satan and his contemporary cousin, nihilism. It's not a credentials race or a contest. I once asked God to save me and the Devil to leave me alone; of course their responses were rather spotty. That taught me more about the futility of begging than about the evidence of spirit. But I never thought sex was a deity, so I searched only for knowledge—looking and touching and thinking it over. That search requires neither faith nor favors, and I've never come away empty.

losing it all

Martyrdom covers a multitude of sins.

Mark Twain

One evening a couple of years ago, I was sitting in a small-town police station three thousand miles from home, waiting in limbo after they cleared the college auditorium where I was supposed to speak. There had been a bomb threat—directed at me. This was a small girls' school in western Massachusetts, where the campus looked like a turn-of-the-century set of dollhouses. With the stars out on a quiet night, and snowflakes falling, I felt like I was inside a little snow globe. Why would anyone want to blow up this delicate toy? One moment I was ready to climb up onto the stage; the next, I was escorted back down by two firefighters who told me we had to evacuate. "Why, where's the fire?" I asked, and they looked surprised, as if I was oblivious to the smoke curling out from under my shoes. "It's you!" one said, leading me to an

equally bewildered police sergeant, who explained that someone had phoned the university and said that a bomb would go
off if I were allowed to speak.

My speech was worth a death threat? My sexual point of view
was that dangerous? I didn't feel like a leader; I felt sick, sorry
for myself. I thought, "If I never see my daughter again, will it
have been worth it just so that I got one last chance to tell some
snooty coeds where their clitoris is?" The more I thought about
my family, the more I cried. I didn't care if the whole town
remained frigid, ignorant, and divided. Let them eat their
dogma soup and choke on it without my assistance. I couldn't
believe I was risking my neck where pagans fear to tread, in
witch-burning country. I felt like a fool, not a revolutionary.

All my life I've seen people who lost what they held dear
because they made the "mistake" of going public—going public,
that is, with something about their sexuality that made people
consider them unfit: unfit for office, unfit for duty, unfit for
family. It's a peculiar word, *unfit*. You are not fitting in, you have
busted all the buttons and ripped out the seams. You must be
removed from all the others who are fitting in. It's as if you have
no island to go to except one with similarly unfit lepers. Even if
you wear your scarlet letter for all to see, it's not punishment
enough to people who are embarrassed and threatened by you;
they simply do not want to see you again. You have fallen, and
everyone hopes that you are so far beneath them now that the
subject will never come up again.

What can I say? I know what beads I rub to inspire myself, I
know what the brave public relations line is. I know that I'm
supposed to tell you about the rewards of honesty and the heroism of sticking your neck out—that this is what makes leaders
instead of sheep. But when leaders are left feeling bitter or,

worse yet, rubbed out altogether, is it worth it? Maybe the sheep are counting their blessings.

Coming out, only to be attacked, is not always intentional. There are so many unlikely and unwilling martyrs who hide from exposure, who want their secrets protected—the opposite of the willing virgin sacrifice. I don't think most people plan to march and die on the cross—they are simply themselves, and that's enough to get them into trouble.

I read a newspaper story about the funeral of young Matthew Shepard, who was murdered in Wyoming by a couple of other young men who found his sexuality a sufficient incitement to beat him to death. At the funeral, yet another young man arrived to picket the burial scene, holding a sign that said, "Go back in your damn closet!" What an ignorant message! Practically everyone does hide in the rear already; most of us choose to stay where we feel comfortable and wanted. Who wants to be criticized and stoned for their most intimate nature? Certainly not the young man who died. He was free to be himself only when he was among like-minded comrades.

A lot of my own willingness to be confrontational comes from the experience of suffering humiliation and discrimination when I wasn't even trying to be noticed, when I was doing my best to fit in. I feel a lot more powerful when I'm the one who initiates the exposure. It's being caught by surprise that leaves me feeling defenseless.

Why would anyone want to blow me up over a message about sex? I've had guns held to my face and my stomach by maniacs who were outraged about trade union activities; I've been stalked by people who, in the name of "Protecting Our Heritage," called me "nigger lover" and left dead rats with their business cards in my bed and at my door. I was frightened terribly by that hatefulness, but in a strange way, I felt prepared for it. I had learned enough of the history of America's racism and labor-management relations to know that both are violent national traditions. But *sex!* There isn't even a word for the act of hating people because they believe in sexual expression. I'd love to use *sexism,* but it's already taken. Why would anyone want to bomb a rally because they resented sexuality? At the police station I felt lonely and wordless, as if I didn't even have an adequate cause.

I told the police captain, "I'm no Martin Luther King, Jr." This fellow was so clean-cut. His hair was shiny black with brilliantine; he had hair on his knuckles and bright-colored pins on his breast pocket. He gave me a look that told me that a comparison with Dr. King had never crossed his mind. I was sitting down, hugging some student's ski jacket over my semi-see-through dress, my tight and festive performing outfit that now was only making me sweat. This officer was unfamiliar with anything having to do with my controversy, and it was embarrassing to answer his questions about the possible identity of this mad bomber.

"Did it sound like a young woman?" I asked, and his eyes brightened.

Aha! "Do you know her then?" he asked. All this would make a lot more sense if it was a family or lovers' quarrel.

"No, but I'm guessing she's a student or alumna from here, probably from the women's studies department." How could I tell this guy what this was all about? I don't think he'd ever attended an elite school like this or lived in a dollhouse. Nobody who goes to these schools becomes a cop. I saw that he wore a wedding band.

"I write and talk a lot about women's sexuality. I think that's what this person is upset about. Some women think that if we are more open about sex, then men will take advantage of us. They think I'm the female Pied Piper of Pornography."

He sized up my explanation. "You're like Dr. Ruth or Gloria Steinem or something," he said. I felt like replying, "No, actually, it's their little protégés that are wishing me dead." But why pout and be sectarian? He was putting it together—one symbol of sexual communication and another icon of women's liberation. Uppity times two.

Freedom for sex and for women—twin ideas that all my life I've thought were worth fighting for. I've always found it righteously easy to agitate for something bigger than our daily bread, something that was worth making a sacrifice for—a connection and transformation bigger than any property, any money, any status. I guess a more conventional patriot would've promoted "public service" or "sacrificing for one's country." I'm not so thrilled with the status quo of my country, so my speeches are a little short on apple pie. But I share the sentiments of any activist who feels that the big picture is what is not only compelling, but necessary. I don't preach the erotic gospel because I'm looking for a hot date.

Then along came my daughter. Families can really kick the shit out of your revolutionary promises. Part of me has resented it, rebelled against it, disinherited it; and yet when I started my own new link, my own child, I felt a protectiveness and cautiousness that I couldn't have dreamed of before. In my dreams I've never refused a risk. Now I have a waking life where I put the brakes on all the time. I used to look at the strangers' faces in a crowd and see the future; now I see the same thing when I look into my daughter's eyes, and I find myself tethered to that vision, her belief in me.

What I realized is that I don't take the risks I do because I'm so noble about my cause, or because my banner of social justice and freedom of expression carries me bodily from issue to issue. No, it's less about revolution in my lifetime and more about revolution in a minute. I get excited and angry and outraged about things—and I just have to say my piece. It's not about saving the world as much as it is about saving my mind. I could shut up, cross my legs, and count my pennies, but I'd be insane before the week was out. I'm not changing the world every minute, but I am protecting my intelligence. I'm not refuting my education. It's just that I'm not getting a lobotomy. I have to use my creativity and outspokenness because it's my way of coping and living and mothering, and of fighting with every daily contradiction. My family is part of this, not separate.

I waited in the police station reading *Boys' Life* for about another hour. Then the same officer came back to me with an offer. "We haven't found anything ourselves in the auditorium, but without a bomb squad search, we can't guarantee your safety in there. The college has offered you the chapel, if you want to speak there instead, or else we should cancel and send everyone home now."

A chapel? He pointed out the station's front window, and I could see it, glowing gold and pink from inside, the prettiest charm in the snow globe. There was a big group waiting outside the station, and I wanted to be with them.

"If it isn't a hoax," he said, "they still would have a hell of a time changing their plans now on the spur of the moment."

I wonder if that was true, or if he just wanted to see me speak himself, from a sermon mount no less. "Let's do it," I said. "I've always wanted to talk about sex from an altar."

My bomber didn't make a second appearance or a phone call. I was on fire at the pulpit, I was hugged in the pews, and I called home the moment it was over to tell my family, "I love you, I love you, this is so insane. . . ."

Why did that young woman who called hate me so much and hide from me? I guessed that she was probably in her late teens, that I was old enough to be her mother. I flashed on one of those tabloid TV programs where a group of indignant young women came on to complain that their moms were all acting like middle-aged sluts. Is this all about feminine envy and competition, after all?.

Women have such a tortured way of showing their displeasure with one another—and it starts so young. My daughter came home from school in tears one day because she got mad at another girl, and her teachers told her that it was wrong to be mad and threatened to expose her anger to me. The type of behavior that they are disciplining in her, as well as in the other girls, shows me that there is, in fact, no way whatsoever that a girl under their watch is allowed to be angry. She can't speak it, she can't write it down in her journal, she can't defend herself. Her "crimes" on these rare occasions are so mild, in terms of their effect, that it's ludicrous. The boys who are her peers would never be punished for such actions. The girls are coached to sit on it, to apologize when they're not really sorry at all.

Instead, the girls, in response, cry and cry and cry; they keep saying, "I'm sorry, I'm sorry, I'm sorry." I feel such bile in my stomach because I know those are tears of anger, the apologies of the oppressed. If they can't express their anger directly, they will soon learn the more "feminine" methods of behind-the-scenes manipulation.

I gave my daughter some contrary advice, which—surprise, surprise—contains elements of sexual awareness and women's liberation. The sexual part amounts to consensuality: if people treat or touch her in a way she doesn't like, she has good cause to insist that they stop. When she expresses her personal feelings in her journal, that's her private space, whether it's hating someone or pouring out her regrets. Her fantasies are not going to go away just because someone else says they're bad. The women's liberation part is my reminding her that the boys argue and resolve hassles with one another every day, and unless it's the rare occasion for an all-out fistfight, none of the grown-ups lifts a finger.

When I get hurt or threatened, when I have terrible regrets—and I do, they haunt me—I can't say anymore, "Oh, I'm *sorry*, watch me cry, because I'm the *sorriest* girl in the world." I had a whole girlhood of being sorry. Maybe I should change the names of my public lectures; instead of saying it's about sex and erotica, I could say, "My talk this evening is about not being sorry." Those who carry bombs may curse me because I have not been bowed, I have not been penitent. The bomb threat vixens are not particularly forgiving anyway; they may be determined to *make* me sorry by hurting as many people as possible. They are like the sadistic Big Sister who wants to see the little girls cry some more, their "sorries" a soaking reminder of their helplessness. I think my hoaxer was well beyond sorriness, and into bitterness and cloaked revenge.

In our world, when people demand an apology they usually want submission, not a renewed spirit. There is, of course, an integrity in a real apology between equals, but how rare a gesture that is! When we are asked to stay closeted, sorry-full, when it is asked of us, "Are you willing to lose everything?" we are actually being asked to keep our spirits in submission indefinitely.

It's the cruelest trick, to hold up everything in the material world that we care about, threatening to take it away—and in the process, leading us to believe that without our "stuff," we have nothing. Since when did bombs make ideas go away? How does scolding children evaporate their desires? How did making sex a sin and an abomination make our creativity disappear?

I don't think I'll ever be prepared for the surprise attack. I'm sure I'll feel fearful and sorry again, I'm sure I'll take a loss. I'll hate every minute of it. But if I have a minute next time, a minute to catch my thoughts, I will know where the fire is. I'll have an answer when the innocent bystanders ask me what the hell is going on. "I'm just like Martin Luther King," I'll say, keeping my face perfectly straight. "I am uppity, and I'm not sorry about it." If anyone asks who's ever been on the spot about being sorry, or whether their penitence is worth losing their freedom, they'll understand why I'm not losing it.

lovers' ethics

A lie can run around the world six times while
the truth is still trying to put on its pants.

Mark Twain

Is there ever a good time to lie
about sex?

Yes, constantly! But when is a bright lie the right idea? And
when should we have the courage to come forth with the more
complicated truth of sexual matters? That's a story that few citizens or lovers are happy to tell.

The fin-de-siècle case of the American president's sexual
affairs brought a good deal of the country to its knees (some on
pads and some on nails) to press our faces to the window of our
standard-bearing role-model, to pronounce him fit or finished.

"Everybody lies some of the time," people say. Aren't we
going to be ashamed of ourselves if we cast the first stone?

I, for one, couldn't help but imagine the worst during the
entire White House scandal, just as I have feared the worst when

I've been caught in my own sexual lies. The reason that the scandal's characters were so compelling on television was because they rang so true to life. Meanwhile, a great many Americans were gasping for air, wishing that someone powerful would show what kind of integrity is possible in one's love life, what a lovers' ethic could be. I dreamed the same dream, but I decided it was impossible with this cast. I can't look for lovers' ethics in the politico's world of double standards and opportunism.

I find more hope just looking around my own community. Who among us hasn't been rocked by a romantic triangle, confronted with the agony of consequences set in motion by the painful truth—or by a risky lie? I've been in all three rotten corners of that triangle myself: the lover who pursued her desire at all costs, the object of that desire, and the one who felt betrayed by the pursuit.

In each case, whether I chose secrecy or confrontation, I did so without a net. There was no perfect standard by which my peers or family judged my actions, only the situation itself.

Oh, sure, I know what my culture's "moral standards" are: a virtual cheesecloth of "Just Say No" incantations. What wouldn't I give for even one politician to get up and say, "One thing I've learned from this awful mess is that we must decriminalize sex between consenting adults"! Now *that* would take some honesty, not to mention balls.

When was the last time any leader came forward to say it's important to affirm the freedom of erotic association and choice? They won't do it because sexuality is what they shame their opponents with. A politician will never tell everyone to fuck off and mind their own business because they do believe it's everybody's business. It's not only some nasty compromise they make, it's a faith. Our political culture believes in sin, and in Madonnas and whores; it believes that sexual pleasure will lead you astray. Clinton bought the compost heap and now he's lying in it.

If our presidents were born-again feminists, instead of preachy Goody Two-Shoes, they would recognize that they are being humiliated for their sexuality. The presidency itself is being made out to be a floozy. Maybe if our virtually all-male Congress had to talk to a few professional whores, they'd get a glimmer of what it's like to be discriminated against for your sexuality every day of the week. But they don't have the first clue about that; their own chauvinism is constantly handing them a rope.

So, fine, let them all hang; but what about the rest of us? Many of us are clear on the kind of sexual politics we'd like to support in public life, but we're still utterly lost when it comes to our own private twisting and turning. There is a huge gap between our sexual lives on paper, as addressed by antiquated laws and puritan punishment, and what real people are going through.

I know what consensual sex is, but sometimes that doesn't help. Once I was hopelessly attracted to a lover who had such violent fits of anger that I wondered whether we'd both live to see the next day. One night in bed, after I'd caught him in a pretty embarrassing lie, he put his hands around my neck and squeezed hard. I couldn't breathe. He looked into my pink eyes and whispered, "If you say one more word—one—I'll kill you." He rolled over and amazingly sank into a deep sleep within seconds. Why didn't I just walk out on that scene immediately? Why wouldn't I tell my friends the truth? Why did I hide what was going on? Eventually my fantasy of the relationship derailed—but was it the truth that finally wised me up, or just sheer scariness?

Other times I've tried the "truth" and hated it. I told some-one I loved as a best friend that I couldn't be a lover to him with-out an erotic attraction; and after that great blast of fresh air, he didn't speak to me again for years. It was agony, and I always had to wonder, "Was I stupid?" Why couldn't I have been more sly, so that it all would have seemed like it was his idea to let things die down?

Another time my lover left me while I was away on a brief summer vacation, but I realized it only because, when I came home, she made love to me but would not let me make love to her. (That was her way of being faithful to her new girlfriend.) I asked, "What's going on? What happened?" and she was com-pletely mute. She never told me a damn thing, and I said to her, "Damn it, if you won't tell me what's going down, I'm going to make it up!" I'll never know how close my made-up story was to the truth, or whether I'm glad she spared me.

We lie with gallantry to protect someone's feelings or reputa-tion, we lie with pragmatism to save face, we lie in fear to avoid conflict, and we lie in loyalty—to at least keep the appearance of a promise.

Underneath those sympathetic emotions, however, we lie to maintain control. If you lie to your lovers to protect their feel-ings, you are first and foremost protecting yourself from their reaction: anger, disappointment, indifference, whatever. If your beloved learns what you are up to, then she or he will be able to react, and you will not control the story.

We value the *appearance* of trust over actual trust; we'd rather pledge monogamy than discuss it. A higher moral standard would place a higher regard on accountability and equality, which in intimate relationships means a greater esteem for trust and truth.

The not-so-noble reason that people lie about sex is less complex. Sometimes it's because it really isn't a big deal. We don't report an occasional one-night stand because we consider it unimportant. Once a woman who had an encounter with my lover approached me in the park, saying, "Don't you want to talk to me about this? Didn't he tell you?"

Yes, he told me, and—not to be rude, but—I forgot about it. He had fun, it was nice, but it didn't change our lives. As a veteran of open relationships, I've learned that while some affairs create unbearable jealousy and insecurity, others just don't have that punch. Maybe you have other fish to fry.

There's a difference between secrecy—hiding significant information—and privacy, which is our right to maintain an existence that isn't constantly orbiting around our mate. Secrecy devastates relationships, but privacy enhances them, because it distinguishes us; it resists the urge to merge.

I know what I've just described may sound unnatural to some. Most Americans I talk to act as if monogamy is God's natural law—but that's what most of the world thought about slavery for centuries as well. Modern monogamy is a combination of our natural tendency to "pair up," chilled by a heavy dose of property rights—"*you belong to me*"—which suppresses our equally natural desire for sexual variety. We do dream of pairing up, of divine and lasting chemistry, but we also wonder what else is out there. The two yearnings are not exclusive.

Sexual desire will have its way with us. We will put on and cast away a hundred masks to disguise it and deny it, but then it will grin at us, strangely unafraid of the consequences. It's become a national joke now to hear politicians rue their "youthful indiscretions," as if tender youth were the cause of it all! Every decade has its own sweet nest of indiscreet opportunity; every year we grow more aware of who we are erotically and of what thrills us or threatens us. Hiding doesn't work, and aging doesn't cover it.

When the president lied about his sexual affairs, he got tattled on; yet even if he hadn't, I doubt that he'd find a lasting peace. In the short term, his public denial must have felt like a huge relief, when he thought his secret was safe. It's the same for millions of Americans who don't relish discussing these kinds of intimate problems any more than Bill Clinton does; they hope their secrets are just as secluded. Out, damn spot! Can't we just get to work on time and leave sex out of it? Yet the harder we deny it, the deeper the mark.

I regret that I did not tell my best friends about my violent lover—not because it would have ensured my leaving him the next day, but because they would have told me similar stories from their own lives, and that would have given me courage.

I wish I had been less clumsy about letting my dear friend down—but I'm glad I was honest. Years later, when even harder things happened, he trusted me, and I love him now more than ever.

As for my lover who left me with no story—when I met her again ten years later, she told me that she couldn't remember anything from that time, because she was always high. I told her my made-up story that I had used to comfort myself, and she said it was a good one to listen to, sober. I was glad to throw it away; I don't need it anymore.

If our political leaders were truthful, and if that truth required tolerance and equality, then it would signal the revolution I've longed for. But that would only be the paper side. A real sexual revolution will never be led by the government; it's the last to respond and the first to defend the most degrading status quo. Our legal and political standards for sex and public policy are

Victorian. We don't have leaders who scrutinize the antiquated moral tyranny—witness Jocelyn Elders, who made one little peep about masturbation, and immediately lost her head by the king's command.

No, it's those in the trenches of lust, unfettered by partisan opportunities, who have been the ones to test honesty, respect privacy, and honor without false pretenses. We're covered in mud, but that's because we're close to the ground. We can only ask ourselves: Where's an army of lovers when you need them?

absolution

When something so wrong feels so right . . ." I've heard that refrain playing in my head since the beginning of my conscious erotic thoughts. It's echoed in so many songs, so many stories—along with its imperative, the bad thing we simply must do. Sometimes I laugh at it, like, what is this, the sociopaths' party joke? Other times I've believed in it and suffered under it like a conviction; living with the humiliation.

Sometimes the grace of knowledge clears up your tragic mis-understanding. There was the time when my formal sex education began, and I could look up a word like *masturbation* and say, "Oh, it wasn't wrong after all; the wrong was in the ignorance, the superstition." For some years I lived with that happy, politically reformed consciousness, where simple things that had been fearsome and sinful became as wholesome as breakfast. Nudity, orgasms, fresh air and exercise, making love under the stars, peppermint tea. How could one find fault in sex when it was Heidi Land: well scrubbed, sweet, putting roses in your cheeks? My mind was at ease . . . except when I was very, very aroused. The things that went through my mind when my clit was on fire were not things that little Heidi could possibly understand.

I didn't understand them, either. I never acknowledged my excesses, my masochism, my voyeurism, my fetishes, my sadism, because those, after all, are the clinicians' descriptions—having to do with the psychos, the lunatics. In my childhood erotic fantasies, my wanderings were not diseased or criminal. My fantasies were the most innocent extension of make-believe stories I'd been telling myself my whole life. I always liked spies and pirates and princesses when I was little—and with that cast of characters, how could I expect anything but eroticism of high drama and danger?

When I was about eight, there was a very popular show called *Get Smart*, and as an adult I can tell you that it was a Mel Brooks satire on Cold War spy politics. However, in my third-grade consciousness, the satire and historical context were all lost on me. I thought it was a funny but scary spy show with all sorts of risqué sexual small talk between the hero, Agent 86, and his girlfriend, Agent 99. Agent 99 was so beautiful to me. Even her name—the number 99—just seemed dripping with sex. I especially liked the opening credits, where the swinging horn music drove our man through a series of doors that kept slamming and opening, alternately claustrophobic and then—POW!—opening up one more escape.

So here's my fantasy. I'm Agent 99—Agent 86 is such a dork, he's out of the picture entirely—and I'm being pursued through those steel doors. If whoever is chasing me catches me, something—POW!—is going to happen to me. Through the pursuer's eyes, watching me, I can see the breathless doe-eyed 99 running, running; but I feel her feelings, that I am going to be trapped, and the unbearable feeling of what will be done to me.

One night the suspense and peril and intrigue of my "99" chase fantasies became *so* suspenseful and *so* intriguing that I came. The steel doors opened, and I fell down my very first rabbit hole. Of course I didn't know I had just had "solo sex," but I did know that I had shattered something, I had pissed all over something, and it was the first thing that had ever made my imaginary scenario stop dead in its tracks. Plus, it wasn't the powerful explosion in my genitals that shocked me back to real-world consciousness, but rather the fact that it stopped. I had pushed that door open a million times in my dreams, and now the fall was as delicious as I had imagined. Only hitting the ground woke me up.

I don't like most of the territory that we have in public for talking about our sexual imagination. Those labels and pro/con banalities make everything I ever dreamed about seem either abnormal or ill fitting. I've already rejected the debates about "normality," with all their attendant pathological and religious bigotries. What's left among the fun seekers and liberals is not all to my liking, either. People ask me, "Are you into S/M?" as if we were talking about a line of cards—my fetish as a consumer dish du jour. I don't buy it—the ethos of "My sexual preference is my lifestyle is my politics is my record label." I feel embarrassed when I'm asked for my label, and it's not for shame about my erotic preferences; it's the stupidity of having my most intuitive and creative moments crammed into sound bites.

Why am I not rejoicing that so many people feel free to joke and make hobbyist conversations about their sexual tastes? After all, they're not tying a noose around their necks in the closet, or subjecting their loved ones to insupportable antics of repression. If Calvin Klein wants to get behind the Kinky Krusade, if Nike wants to court erotic chic in athletic advertisements, who am I to wax nostalgic over the days when we whispered to ourselves like fugitives? But I don't think I'm nostalgic for the bad old days; I'm finding the current liberal definitions insufficient. We're still dealing with sex like it was an eight-crayon box.

What color am I, after all? I champion the rights of leather-hood or whatever-hood, but I'm crap as a poster child. I'm a poor example of an S/M vixen if the definition has to do with how many torture devices I have at my disposal (the average kitchen has more than enough) or how many knots I've learned to tie.

But, suppose you ask me: Have I ever become aroused by thoughts of pain, of unbearable endurance, of forced confessions and impossible cruelties? Have I found objects entertaining? Have I taken my impatience and turned it into a sensation-filled punishment? Have I broken every family and social taboo with obscene screams and lustful begging? I'll nod my head like a not-so-dumb animal.

I have entertained the *un*-wholesome, the anti-Heidi. I am secure in my faith that others have had similar thoughts and that we walk among one another not knowing, oblivious. It's only when I have time to reflect, like during commercial TV breaks or in a car at the red light, that I think about how closely guarded we keep our erotic identities. How many of my comrades-in-thought-crimes have acknowledged their imaginations or discussed their fantasies with even one other person? I can only get depressed at what a tiny minority that might be.

As popular as analysis and self-transformation may be in our culture, as much as we drag every bit of wretched violence and neurosis out of our family and institutional closets, the fact that these things exist in our sexual world, in our erotic thoughts, is something most people think of as sad or danger-ous. We think, even if we're unafraid of it ourselves, that people will take our sexual thoughts *the wrong way*. They'll think we're tragic, we're suffering from a lack of fiber or the absence of a mother's love.

I'm not sad and I'm not brutal. I know that every shade of sexual emotion is what makes the juice of eroticism. There is no orgasm that is as lightweight as soapsuds, there is no erotic energy that isn't heavy, that floats with no sting. I appreciate Muhammad Ali's metaphor about the butterfly and the bee because it speaks so well about sex.

I don't think actual "kinky" sex is as frightening to the public as the titillation of its discovery. We are led to expect a grisly result, the punishment and horror of the deviant thought. It doesn't matter whether one person's version of kinky is chains and candle wax, while another person is contemplating simple vanilla homosexuality—the fears are the same.

"Oh, Tom, I'm so frightened, I think Pat might be *that* way!"

"Oh, no, Susan, you don't mean *that* way, do you? We've got to get Pat some *help* before it's too *late!*"

Yes, Pat-the-Pervert is not an accurate description of any-one's real life but is, rather, the medical and sometimes crimi-nal label that leaves us no room to be anything but professional deviants. A label is a quick and sticky way to calm the concerns of the conforming womb. What lies outside Vanilla Land? "Pat"

knows, but we're led to believe Pat won't even make it out alive.
Don't we treat people like that with drugs or lock them up or in
some effective way just take them out of circulation? We're
confident that the Pats of the world won't tell on themselves if
we deny their existence. We are warned away from pleasure
and self-discovery like children being told not to look in a
cupboard.

Yes, there are always do-gooders who seek to justify their
fears of the sexually unfamiliar. They point to the scary incarcer-
ated offenders, the serial whatevers, and say: How do we control
people like *that*, who took their sick little fantasies and hurt
someone?

Right then, we feel like we should be roused to action; we've
got to *stop* the erotic fantasies because somebody somewhere
might *do* something—and yet you can see where this kind of
logic gets you. We don't try to stop people from *thinking* about
anything except sex, no matter how heinous their future crimes
might be. Why do we think eroticism is the problem in crimes
where the most compelling inhumanity is not the sex, but rather
the complete lack of compassion? Instead of asking, "Why are
you attracted to X?" we should be asking, "Why don't you have
any empathy? How come you don't see where you *end* and someone else *begins*?"

But let's put all that aside for a minute. No one writes a
gourmet cookbook and spends most of its pages addressing food
poisoning. No one edits a magazine about cars and fills its text
with gory warnings about accidents. Why should I write a book
about eroticism and devote myself to a vale of sex fears?

Behind every anxiety about sexual violence is a much deeper
predation: fear of pleasure, fear of righteous pleasure, fear of
powerful pleasure. Fear of hands that know their sexual body so

well that they grow hair. Fear of a lust that would make women demanding and men weak in the knees. What every citizen understands about kinky sex, if they don't know a single other detail, is that this deviation, whatever it is, is somehow making sex more intense and more pleasurable. Someone is going to the moon on these sensations, someone is risking everything to feel it again. And it's this extreme and sought-after rocket to ecstasy that offends us so—not fear at all, but suspicion and envy in spades.

electricity

Last summer, through a series of lucky accidents, I hosted an old-school bluegrass band overnight at my house, following its local debut. They were from South Carolina, had never been to California before, and had only a dim idea of what I do for a living. The drummer was particularly interested in what I had in my library, and before he left I gave him a suitcase of all my books on sexual politics, covering everything from anal intercourse to the Supreme Court. I didn't know if I'd hear from the band again, but he wrote me a month later when they landed back home. "I really liked reading your books on the road," he said, "and there's so many things I'd like to talk about. But let me just ask you this for now: Have you ever experienced electricity during sex?"

For a moment I flashed on the sensory memory of a burning smell between my sheets the time my vibrator shorted out under my bedcovers. But I knew that he wasn't talking about that, a truly rarefied experience. No, I think he meant something that happened while making love, a current between him and his lover.

I was curious that my new friend didn't define what he meant by "electricity." He didn't say, "Have you ever been really in love? Have you ever felt another presence?" When people feel an unexpected or extrasensory jolt during sex, they typically chalk it up to true love or a sign from their god. It is usually interpreted as a romantic signal that you are with the "right" person doing just the "right" thing—although a few people who have been around the block will admit that sparks are capable of flying even with people they know they couldn't spend eight hours with, let alone the rest of their lives.

The other curiosity about sexual "electricity" is that it makes such a powerful impression that many people who report the sensation will describe with awe that they weren't even touching genitals, stoking the conventional orgasm.

I first became interested in this sort of electricity when I was learning about the sexual reeducation of lovers who had spinal cord injuries or paralysis that made their genital area numb. One of the most erotic films I have ever seen was a documentary for couples where one lover has a spinal cord disability. On cam-era, these couples had undeniably powerful and expressive sex. The last thing I expected to feel, watching a documentary about sex for the disabled, was envy, but that's exactly what I was left with. The camera didn't show any white lightning, the screen didn't crackle, but with one couple in particular, I felt like their every touch was completely off the ground.

I know people seek this kinetic experience, avidly, by study-ing books and applying themselves to meditation, prayer, or exhaustive searches for the complete and perfect partner. However, some of the most impressive stories I've heard about electricity were in situations that were anything but high-minded or spiritually considered. Why do some people get their first jolt at a billiard parlor, when others are in a temple? If you feel it once with someone, why not forever, why not every time?

I cannot describe for you the chemistry of sexual electricity, though I have certainly had open ears to all scientific, paranormal, and spiritual explanations. The one thing I am convinced of is that these bolts of body thunder are neither romantic halos nor fortune-telling advisories. They do, however, convey a sense of possibility and invention where there was nothing before, a seamless cloth. This electricity is not something you only feel when looking into the eyes of a lover; it's a catalyst that can happen when you are alone—maybe a song that deeply moves you or even a spell of strong weather that brings out something in you that you can't explain. It can touch you in a crowd—in chaos, for that matter.

I read a recent newspaper editorial against teenage sexuality, in which a pregnancy prevention counselor explained with great gravity that the reason sexual activity is so seductive to young people, the reason it is so hard to break them from that desire, is that sex gives them such "high self-esteem." She delivered this verdict grimly.

Yes, sexual success does give you high self-esteem. It's so electric that it could probably make your hair stand on end if you found enough people feeling it simultaneously. In a world where self-esteem has become such a cheap cliché, sex is one place where people feel, if only for a short while, that they are powerful, that they are desired and desiring. No wonder it's such an emboldment to teenagers, who typically feel their power thwarted at every turn. A different consciousness rules the air when you feel sexually confident—and it feels like magic.

What's magical is not a rabbit in a hat, or true love in the personal ads. It's our ability to be creative in a world where we feel generous even though our institutions are tight and unforgiving, where we see beauty and pain without the benefit of pointers and price tags.

Does this mean that all these electric lovers, who have had excellent sex and top-drawer climaxes, are smarter and smell better and have whiter teeth? No, it means they have a powerful creative capacity that can be ignited by sexual excitement. More touching and more lovemaking will doubtless feel good to the source of that current, but that's only the beginning. When someone tells me their electric sex story, I don't think, "Oh, you hot stud, you wench"; I think, "What does it feel like to know you could do anything?" Sexual electricity isn't the living end—it's a side effect of what it's like to live with an endless imagination; it's the burn of a memory that just won't quit.

I've had every sort of supernatural sensation in my dreams, my magnificent night life, but I have not experienced a live-wire jolt in my waking moments. I have felt metaphorically on fire when the power of sexual attraction was upon me, but I haven't actually seen any lightning come out of my fingertips.

Well, maybe one time: When I was a young woman, about a year into my adult sex life, I had a married lover who I was mad for. I thought about making love with him night and day. One morning, a few months into it, he told me that our affair was over, as of that minute. He announced it like a military briefing—one sentence, no questions.

We were alone preparing a room for a meeting, and I was unfolding chairs. I kept unfolding them, one row after the next. He was up in front fiddling with the podium.

"Plug in that lamp," he said, pointing to a loose cord on the floor near my foot.

I picked up the prong end and pressed it into the wall outlet, only to get the shock of my life—blue sparks, smoke, and a jolt that went from my fingertips to my jaw. I cried out; tears poured out of my eyes and burned my face almost as badly as the electric shock had scorched my arm.

He flew to my side and picked me up off the floor. "I'm sorry, baby, please, I'm so sorry," he said. I couldn't see his eyes. He held me in his arms, he opened a button of my shirt and buried his head in my chest. My arm was still shaking. I could feel his erection through my jeans, I could feel him pressing against me. "This is so fucked up," I thought. I was so turned on. The affair did not end as of that minute.

In my dreams afterward, I was in the same place again, and the current spiraled from my palms to my nipples to my cunt to the wall. I was sopping wet when I woke up. Right there, that deep blue shock, is the closest I've ever come to electricity during sex.

roll your own erotic manifesto

> In revolution, as in a novel, the most
> difficult part to invent is the end.
>
> Alexis de Tocqueville

I. Talk about sex anywhere.

The most audacious act of public sex is talking about it. Sex is as delicious a conversation piece as food or music; it is as infinite as weather, and twice as interesting. Sexual conversation puts an end to small talk and small minds. It belongs at dinner tables and airports and church, and anywhere that people exchange ideas.

Some people think that sex talk is gossip—that it's a rude joke, a calculated play. Maybe they've never had a talk about sex that was honest, or that ended with a question mark, or that was intellectual and even luscious. Maybe they've never talked about sex without a threat underlying it.

What could you say about sex today, to a friend or stranger, that would open the doors, instead of shutting someone out?

II. Take inspiration from everyone and instruction from no one.

You never have to worry about becoming a sexual imitation of someone else, because it's impossible. You only have to worry when you hide your true side, your fear at the thought of showing your joy at what delights you, or your despair when silence seems like the only way to survive. Erotic creativity is like a modern dancer—she has a body, she listens to the music, she takes a deep breath, and she *moves*. No one can tell her which foot goes first, or how to bend. The erotic spirit listens and expresses, never memorizes or recites.

III. Appreciate the simplest erotic gesture.

The headiest erotic memories are from times never advertised, from moments that could not be packaged. Genuine beauty will arrive with great modesty, and yet with a perfection that cannot be reproduced in facsimile. Of course we want to make these moments last, we dream of manifesting them as jewels. But the pleasures of possession are so fleeting. It is the treasure of your sexual creativity, combined with your lover's imagination, that makes erotic flavor last.

IV. Accept no guru's ego—accountability is more cosmic than charisma.

The greatest gift that leaders can give to their followers is the opportunity to disagree with them, to have a vote, to remain a comrade despite disagreement. There are no sexual gurus who know how to make your erotic body happy with their philosophies, and there never will be any. The best sexual adviser is the person who is the best listener, who asks the best questions, and more than anything, who appreciates the chance to be fallible in public.

V. Give your erotic identity the benefit of your admiration.

I have never been able to post positive affirmations on my mirror. I can't abide those personal exercises where you look at your reflection and say, "I'm fabulous and that's that." I could never resist the notion that such speeches are all the latest trick from Snow White's wicked stepmother.

But I am not entirely filled with piety and humility. I do talk to myself—without notes or reflective surfaces. Sometimes I look at my eyes in the mirror and think about how the fire there is always going to be in there no matter how old I get.

The best thing that ever happened to my sex life was when, by accident, I stopped making comparisons to others—when I was momentarily distracted, and just let myself think and make love as I am. I was at my most content and my most thrilled. If I had happened to catch a glance of myself in the mirror, I would have been surprised—because when I am involved in life, my activity animates my face and body in a way that could never be caught in a pose.

VI. Defy the quick description.

Next time someone asks you what you "are," sexually, tell them that nouns will not do. Deliver a story of the last time you were sexual, or imagined an erotic fantasy; and this description will be full of verbs and adjectives and even material that almost defies words. You may have to show it with your hands. Labels, every one of them, should be saved strictly for protest signs and sandwich boards.

VII. Kill envy with erotic kindness.

Envy will wrap around you like a vise—and in its grip you will fear that you will lose, that you don't have a chance. You will circle the ones whose lives you covet, hexing them or vexing yourself, but you won't touch the fire in the middle.

Envy needs an *un*-Convention to vanquish its tenacity. The opposite of envy isn't carelessness, it's compassion, and we need to cherish it. Instead of feeling smug or angry in your envy, you can start tasting your own fear. Only gentleness and forgiveness will allow that frightful taste to dissolve. Why can't we tell people how we really feel about sex? Why can't we consider our erotic imagination? It's not because someone else has possession of it.

VIII. Claim your own fantasy life. Write it all down, every bit of it.

Many people do not think that they have fantasies, or they believe their fantasies cannot be articulated. Others think their fantasy lives are so banal that it is easier to refer to a few generic descriptions. But whether you think you are fantasy-free or a walking stereotype of cheesy porn, if you actually recorded your aroused thoughts in detail, you would find you are neither.

As my friend Jack Morin says in *The Erotic Mind*, "Imagine yourself really wanting to be sexually aroused and for some reason you're not. Based on everything you know about your sexuality, describe the fantasy that would be the very most likely to arouse you."

IX. Make a recipe for fantasy revelation.

Masturbate. Tell yourself before you begin that you are going to track your thoughts and remember them, much as you might do before you go to bed, telling yourself that you want to remember your dreams. When you begin to get aroused, observe your thoughts without judgment or self-conscious comment.

Right after you orgasm, as if after a dream, reach for a pen and paper next to you, and write down every detail you remember. Describe the climax of the fantasy—not your body necessarily—at the most intense point of your erotic thoughts. Once you have written a fantasy recipe, read it out loud and you will hear something that will surprise you in a most illuminating way.

X. Describe a sexual experience you've never had.

Imagine the taboo, the physically impossible, the offensive, and the just plain surreal. Become an erotic mind traveler with great glee and boundless tolerance. Let yourself be infected with others' sexual charisma—even if you'd never do what they do in a million years. Of course you wouldn't! Erotic mimicry is hopeless—what's possible, and pleasurable, is appreciation and curiosity.

If you can't empathize with sexual inspiration from unpredictable sources, you are turning a deaf ear to your own imagination, and your creativity will suffer more than you can measure.

XI. Decloak right in the middle of fucking.

Expose yourself. Say out loud what you're thinking.

For the longest time, I didn't know that sex talk was an instant aphrodisiac. I would write about sex, I would speak publicly and most graphically—but in bed, I would never voice a word of my fantasies. With longtime lovers, this became even more inexplicable, since I shared so many other things with them, private fears and embarrassments. How could saying my sexual wishes out loud be so catastrophic, when they knew everything else? I was like one of those people who won't let her picture be taken. My erotic voice was my great secret, and I felt like my orgasm would be lost forever if I opened my trap.

My friend Lisa Palac was the catalyst in coaxing my erotic voice box out of its hiding place. She produced a record called *Cyborgasm*, an album of various people's erotic stories. She asked to tape one of mine. I wasn't to describe it as an impartial observer—recording the "pillow talk" was supposed to be as hot as if it were entirely private.

I closed my eyes in front of the mike. I had never told a story so vividly. At the end, I realized that my fantasy did not seem in the least diminished—I felt high, in fact. At that point, I guess you could say I was provoked into going home and giving it a try with one very surprised lover.

XII. Make your own pornography, accept no imitation.

If you don't like what you see out your window, the most subversive and substantive thing you can do is to make your own vision. If criticizing sex is so important, then where are our role models? Who do you think is going to make erotic expression meaningful to you if not yourself?

Write your own story, your own lyric, pick up the camera. Stop arguing about what is erotic or pornographic, and show me the transcendental sensation. Technology has put the erotic power of any production into the hands of lovers—why not use it?

XIII. Never apologize as a submissive.

Forgiveness and humility are unusual and welcome graces. We are more accustomed to subservience, helplessness, and swallowing bile, all under the guise of "I'm sorry." Genuine sorrow is a different emotion than being sorry-full. The gift of taking responsibility is a bouquet, it's the opposite of a thousand regrets. Don't tell me you're sorry when you're angry, or when you're horny, or when you're indifferent. That's a wound, not a realization.

XIV. Teach your children privacy, in all its aspects, not just sexual.

Our kids do not belong to us, as tempting as that might be to think. Our memory that they came out of us is misleading because they are not our words, our thoughts, or our waste. They have their own imaginations that we neither create nor undo; they live in our house, but they have their own world. We can respect and admire their world by giving them privacy, tolerance, an appreciation for our own bodies, and a great feeling of love beyond possession.

XV. Expose your body to the sensuous elements.

Appreciate weather, from sheets of rain to winter sun to twilight humidity. Firelight, candlelight, spotlights, light of all kinds. Other people's skin, their face, their genitals, their hair around your fingers. Baby skin, and feather-soft old people's skin. Large balls of softness, and edges that might be too sharp. Things that melt in your mouth and your hands. Anything that stings. It's all pure balm.

XVI. Assume everyone is sexual.

To ever imagine otherwise is one of the most profound and ignorant forms of discrimination.

> Your momma is sexual,
> Your great-grandma who you never even knew,
> Her husband too—
> Your precious baby, and every other precious baby,
> That twisted-up guy in a wheelchair,
> The thirteen-year-old with thick glasses and
>   orthopedic shoes,
> The incredibly homely person that you crossed the
>   street to get away from,
> weird anorexic supermodels too—
> Anyone you don't desire,
> and anyone you've ever put on a pedestal.
> EVERYONE